AF441805

WHY SUFFER
WITH A BAD BACK?

WHY SUFFER WITH A BAD BACK?

commonsense and practical advice on treatment of disorders of the lower back

Peter Baranowski M.D., Sp.N., Dp.Chir.
(Leningrad, Berlin, Munich)

ANGUS & ROBERTSON PUBLISHERS

Angus & Robertson Publishers
London • Sydney • Melbourne • Singapore • Manila

First published by Angus & Robertson Publishers, Australia,
1980

National Library of Australia
Cataloguing-in-publication data.

Baranowski, Peter.
   Why suffer with a bad back?

   ISBN 0 207 14172 x Hardbound
   ISBN 0 207 14139 8 Paperbound (available only in the U.K.)

   1. Backache. I. Title.

616.7'3'06

Printed in Hong Kong

To my patients, and to all Australians
I dedicate my book

*I wish to express my sincere thanks to my
daughter Tania without whose time and effort
this book would not have appeared in the
English language*

Contents

Illustrations

Doctor's Report

This means a foreword by another doctor. Only an accident of his wanderings prevented Peter Baranowski from ornamenting the Australian medical profession. So he has worked here as a health professional outside the club and succeeded by his wisdom instead of by his diplomas.

The word wisdom is carefully chosen. As you read this book you will realise that it is not the work of a young man. It does not transmit cheap knowledge culled from other men's writings; it deals in personal conclusions acquired critically in the consulting room.

It cares nothing for current fashion. It promises no quick successes and sells no magic formulae. It outlines the methods and principles of the reputable rheumatic spas and hydropathic institutions which flourished in Europe between the wars. These are rationalised by newer learning and modified by years of experience in a busy clinic serving an accident-prone farming community.

It is clearly written for the intelligent, non-medical reader. The further you read the more practical it becomes.

In an age in which the technical professions delight in hiding their secrets under mountains of jargon it is a literary delight to follow the author's deft use of a language he acquired during the middle years of his career.

Gordon Leslie, M.R.C.P. (Lond), B.M., B.Ch. (Oxon)
Albany Western Australia 1978

Preface

I was a strong healthy young man and in the near future I was to receive my doctor's degree, something for which I had studied so long and with great enthusiasm. It was a dream of my life to be a doctor.

It had been hard at times, but the goal was in sight.

But, as it sometimes happens, an incident occurred which had a life-long effect on me and, because of that incident, nearly fifty years later this book was "born".

I had come from a lecture and a friend from the same faculty took me aside and whispered in my ear. "Come to the same place tonight where we met last time. You won't be sorry. In fact you'll enjoy it. Bring your notebook because we want you to read some of your poetry and you know how the girls love that."

I had been writing poetry since my earliest school days and it is always very satisfying to have an opportunity to show off one's talent, especially to the opposite sex.

The basement which was our usual meeting place was noisy and smoke-filled when I arrived last and it was apparent that they were waiting for me. My friend stood up and announced, "The poet has arrived! Give him a drink."

I took the proffered glass and was in the act of sitting down on one of the old chairs which were part of the basement's attraction when someone on my left, with more high spirits than sense, pulled the chair from under me and I fell onto the concrete floor, still clutching my glass.

Everyone laughed uproariously, including myself.

My bottom was sore and from time to time as I read a sharp pain like an electric shock would flash through my tailbone and lower back. At these moments my voice grew involuntarily louder as I was reading my poetry.

The happy crowd, by now mildly intoxicated, thought I was reading with increased enthusiasm, not realising that it was pain that added force to my tone.

A few more glasses of wine and vodka helped to dull the pain and I was able to enjoy my evening as much as everyone else, forgetting about the chair that was pulled from beneath me and the idiot who had done it.

I remembered the incident and the "friend" only later on when the spinal pain from which I was to suffer for the rest of my life, started to recur in earnest.

I began my working life at the age of thirteen as a messenger boy in the office of a maternity hospital. However I was sacked a few weeks later because of my determination to know about everything, which the authorities called "curiosity". No doubt they termed it "impertinent" curiosity. Still I did other work. Then I was cleaner and messenger boy again.

During all my teenage years circumstances made it necessary for me to earn my own living and I attended night school classes which always finished very late at night.

As a young man I was a labourer, an orderly in a hospital, a clerk, a physical training instructor and a teacher in medical schools, before I finally began to practise as a doctor. Everywhere, even amongst the smallest group of people with whom I lived, worked and studied, or whom I later observed and treated, were people suffering with spinal troubles.

There is one school of thought that expounds the theory that the life of every individual is charted in advance and that one is powerless to alter one's destiny. I don't know. Perhaps this is so but *I* am not a fatalist.

Perhaps it was fate that a young hooligan pulled a chair from beneath me and damaged my spine so that, suffering the effects for the rest of my life, I should finally decide to write this book so that fellow sufferers might gain some benefit and learn from my misfortune.

Who knows!

Introduction

The accumulated knowledge and wisdom of people of all nationalities have given birth to many cures for the ills with which men are afflicted.

"Less understanding is the doctor who has never been ill himself." In this book the experiences of fifty years have been collected and material has been gathered from medical articles written by doctors in other countries.

Most of my reading, my work, and my concern during those years was directed towards the suffering from, the prevention of and the treatment for spinal disorders. My knowledge and experience has been gained from my work in different countries, with people of many nationalities, of all ages and both sexes. There have literally been thousands of such people.

Because of my own personal suffering I feel I have been able to understand their problems with more clarity. I have been able to sympathise and, above all, advise, because I have had the "doubtful advantage" of being one of their number.

Perhaps, in addition, this book may prevent spinal suffering.

As a doctor specialising in neurology I have had the opportunity, in hospitals and clinics in different countries, to observe and treat patients suffering with problems of the spinal column — especially with the column's roots and nerves.

In this book I have deliberately attempted to make the text as simple and clear as possible, minimising the use of medical and scientific terms which are confusing and often unintelligible to the non-professional reader. This is not a book for members of the medical profession. It is written for the men, and women in all walks of life who are searching for help with their various spinal disorders. This book is for everyone. I have concentrated on being helpful without being dull. I have tried to be comprehensible and, I hope, sympathetic.

Above all, I want this book to be beneficial or my purpose

in writing it will have failed. This book is for everyone but particularly for the ordinary man and for all those people whose work in life may lead them more readily into physical acts that may affect and damage the spine. I feel that I shall have succeeded with this book if my observations of suffering and the experiences of half a century can be used by others who, like me, suffer the unhappy results of spinal injury.

CHAPTER 1

What we know about the spinal column and the spinal cord

Let us be honest and admit that most of us know very little, in fact almost nothing, about our spinal column or spinal cord.

Facts we learned at school have long since been forgotten. Many of us know very little about the complex and wonderful piece of machinery that is our body.

There are many books published today for the man in the street which deal with heart attacks (the modern scourge of the Western world), with arthritis, diabetes, dieting, alcoholism, the harmful effects of smoking, beauty care and sex.

But is there a simply written text book which can tell the ordinary person about the anatomy and physiology of the backbone and spinal cord and what can happen when one sustains an injury to the lower part of the spinal column? Perhaps this is because there are so many different kinds of illnesses in this area and there is a lack of knowledge about how to prevent them.

But we need to know how to *treat* such an injury, how to *prevent* such injuries and how to make the entire backbone more resistant to all kinds of harmful influences, both internal and external.

Man, like all animals, has a skeleton to protect the delicate and complicated internal organs which sustain life. The head and spinal cord, the lungs and heart, are all protected from injuries which may happen and to which they are liable in the daily course of living.

Muscles, ligament and cartilage, together with the bony structure of the skeleton, form a complex system of levers which allow the most diverse and often extremely complex movements. There are more than four hundred skeletal muscles in the body. They are responsible for the movement of the joints, maintenance of posture, support of body weight, circulation of blood, respiration and elimination.

You have only to watch acrobats, sportsmen or dancers to see this complexity illustrated to the highest degree.

There are many bones in the human skeleton but few of us know exactly how many there are and what changes can occur in a person's spine from birth to old age. The human skeleton consists of two hundred and six bones, more than in any other animal on earth, and it is the most perfectly formed of all creatures.

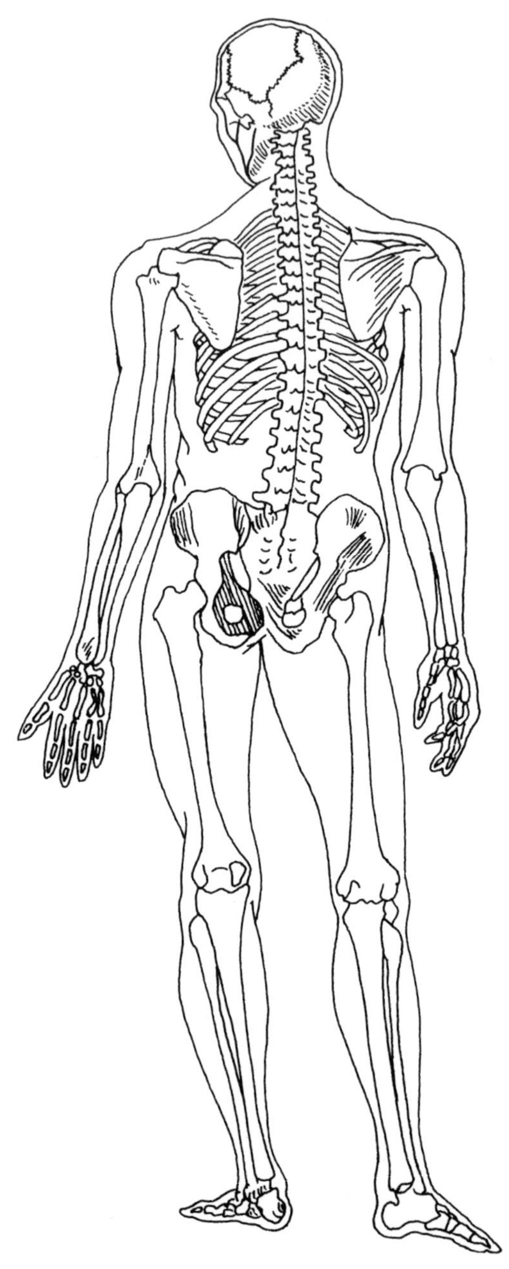

1. The normal human skeleton

The spinal column itself is comprised of 33 or sometimes 34 bones, and the length of it varies according to the height of each person but it is, on an average from 70 to 90 centimetres long.

The spinal column is the main support for the whole body. Without it, we would bend, not only with the burdens we carry but under our own body weight. In fact, without the spinal column we would not be able to walk upright and would have to crawl. It is entirely due to the spinal column that man can remain in a vertical position.

Let us examine how the spinal column is built and why certain parts of it are especially susceptible to injury and disease.

As we have already said there are 33 or 34 bones, called vertebrae, which together form the support for the whole body. This support is our spinal column. It is divided into five parts:

1. The neck, consisting of seven vertebrae, called the cervical area.

2. The chest, consisting of twelve vertebrae, called the thoracic or dorsal area.

3. The lumbar region consisting of five vertebrae, called the lumbar region or, more commonly, the lower back (spine).

4. The sacrum consisting of five vertebrae, called the sacrum.

5. The tail-bone, made up of five, or sometimes only four, undeveloped vertebrae that have joined together into one bone called the coccyx. This is called the coccygeal region.

The vertebrae from which the spinal column is built are not all the same. They are solid at the base but as they approach the skull they become smaller in size and weaker. Vertebrae sit firmly, one upon the other forming a saddle joint. Between every joint there is an elastic cartilage called a disc. Discs give vital and necessary mobility and elasticity but very often they are the reason for great suffering.

Children are born with a stick-like spinal column but during the course of the first years of life, the spinal column changes and develops three curves which are a necessary part of every mature spinal column. The first curve, the neck, is formed in children when they learn to hold up their heads. The second curve is the chest curve (backwards) which is formed when children begin to sit up. The backbone curve, the last curve of the developed spinal column, is formed when children stand upright and learn to walk.

This last curve is the most important of all as it is at this point that the processes of deterioration can begin which may cause great suffering and sometimes may even make someone an invalid.

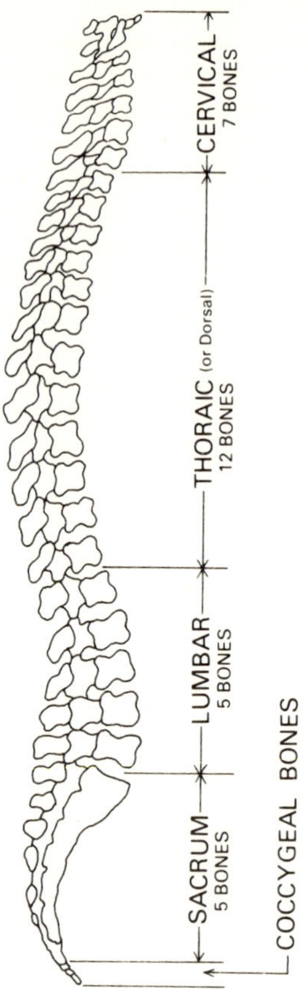

2. Section through the vertebral column

Thanks to the curves and the twenty-three inter-vertebral discs, the spinal column is, to a certain extent, an "absorber" apparatus. Shocks, bumps and all possible shakes are transmitted to it during walking, running, jumping and falling. All the vibrations are weakened and extinguished in its springy mechanism. It is not difficult to understand what an important and protective role the spinal column plays, not only for the spinal cord and its roots hidden in the column, but for all the internal organs of the human body. In fact, the health of the whole body is being protected.

The sacrum and the tail bone form the end of the spinal column. From the age of fifteen to sixteen years, the five single vertebrae of the sacrum begin to grow together and by the age of twenty-five they have already formed one massive three-angled bone. This bone covers the pelvis from the rear and in this way protects from harm the important and delicate urino-genital organs.

The importance of the sacrum bone can be judged from its historic name — *os-sacrum,* which means sacred bone. In ancient times the Druids, during the time of sacrifice, cut out the sacrum from their sacrificial victims. The officiating priest took for himself the best meat which lay behind the sacrum. The sacrum itself was burnt as an offering to the gods.

The last portion of the spinal column is called the os-coccygis. This comes from the Greek word meaning cuckoo and was so named because the ancients saw the tail-bone as resembling the beak of the cuckoo. It is an interesting though not a large bone. Like the sacrum, the tail-bone consists of four or sometimes five undeveloped joint vertebrae. In addition, the last and smallest part of it is often independent. Some scientists think it is really the last vestige of the tails we once had in the early stages of evolution when our forebears were swinging from trees as our monkey "relatives" still do.

So — the spinal column consists of a row of vertebrae sitting one upon the other and in some parts joined together, in the sacrum and tail-bone. All the vertebrae are strongly joined by ligaments and discs. A disc consists of fibrous cartilage tissue. However this is not the complete picture of the complex construction and function of the spinal column.

On the back of each person are distributed the largest and strongest muscles which are all closely connected to the spinal column. There are three kinds of muscles: the superficial, the deep, and the very deep, some of which run from the back of the head to the tail-bone. Each muscle begins and ends with a tendon to which the muscle is joined.

Muscles and tendons of the back in their permanent function hold the spinal column in a straight vertical position. However, their function does not end here. Not only do they give the spine its upright position but they bring the entire spinal column into movement.

Weak spinal muscles and tendons are not capable of supporting the spinal column in an upright position and people begin to stoop. This occurs in the old or the physically weak.

In a young and normal spine, practically all types of movement are possible — bending forward as well as sideways, and straightening up. In the lower region, even a certain amount of rotation is possible. But of all the parts of the spinal column, the neck region is the most flexible and mobile.

In the spinal column, effectively hidden and protected by the vertebrae, is a long and rounded strand, which is one of the most important organs, after the brain. It is also one of the most mysterious and wonderful constructions of the body. It is the spinal cord and it is irreplaceable.

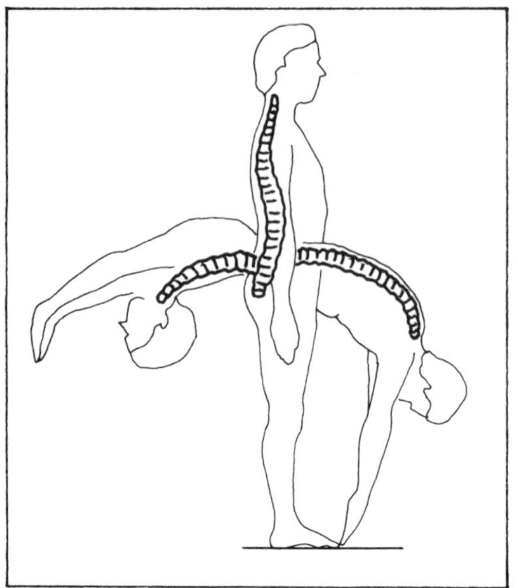

3. *Normal movements in lumbar region*

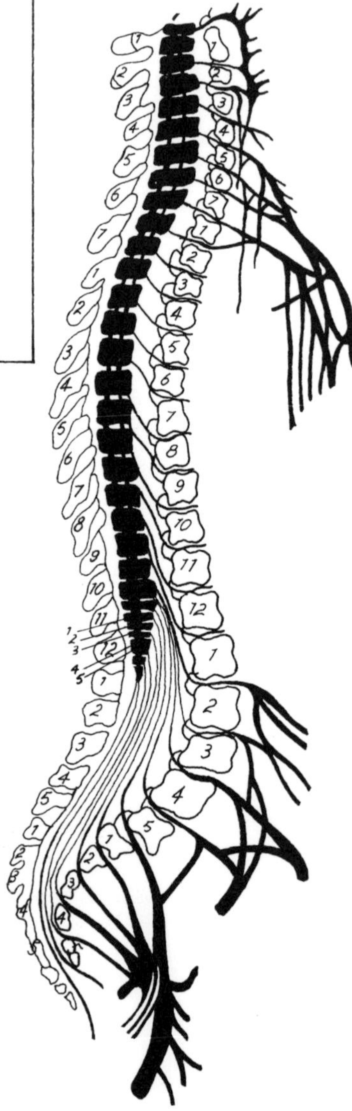

4. *Spinal cord and its position in spinal column*

The spinal cord is approximately 45 centimetres long and its weight in an average person is between 35 and 40 grams. Its thickness is equal to the little finger and only in the lower and upper parts, i.e. the neck and lumbar regions, does it become thicker.

Zoologists have established that where some part of the body is used more than another, the width of the spinal cord is affected. Animals with long limbs have noticeably thicker spinal cords where the limbs begin. For example, the kangaroo uses, primarily, its legs and tail for movement and support. The tail has an especially large widening of the lumbar region of the spinal cord. In orangutans and gibbons, both of which possess very long arms which they use more than their legs, there is a strong thickening of the spinal cord in the neck region.

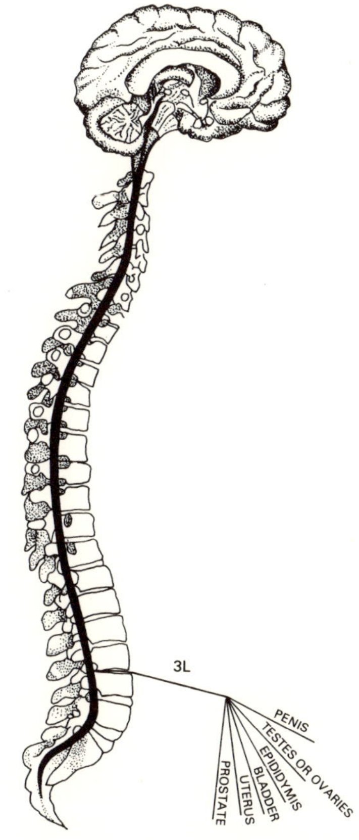

5. Parts influenced by the third lumbar nerve

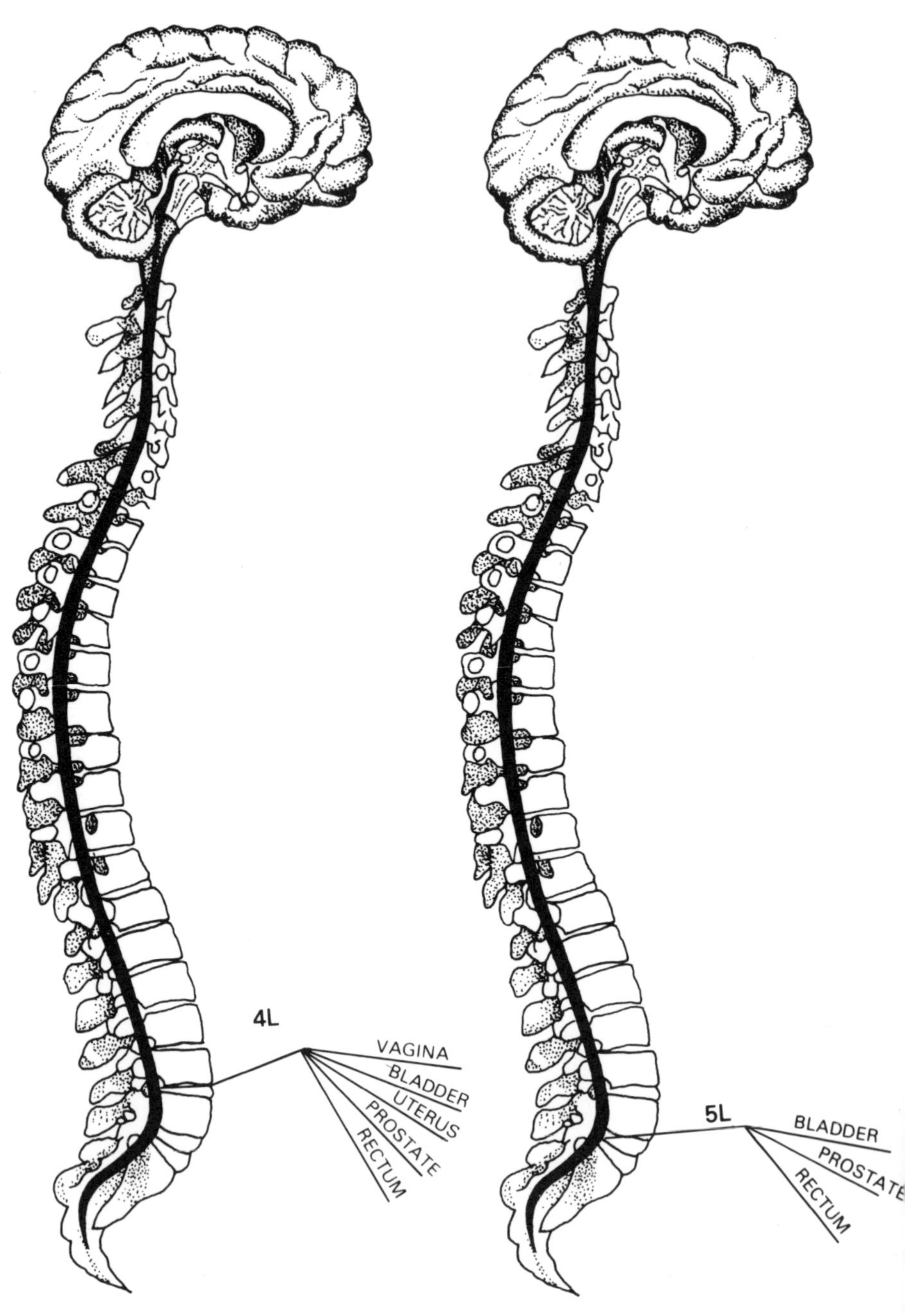

6. *Parts influenced by the fourth lumbar nerve*

7. *Parts influenced by the fifth lumbar nerve*

The spinal cord ends in a bundle of nerves in the lumbar sacrum region of the spinal column and this is called "the horse's tail". Thirty-one pairs of nerve roots leave the side of the spinal cord and they form thirty-one spinal roots on the left and right hand sides. From these roots branch a large number of stems which connect not only with the muscles, but to all the organs of the body. These nerves carry out continuous commands from the brain and regulate the normal function of all the organs of the body, including the heart and reproductive systems.

From the facts so far mentioned concerning the anatomy and physiology of the spinal column and spinal cord and its nerves, it is not difficult to imagine what an enormous role it plays in the life of each person. Nor can one fail to visualise or understand that sometimes irreversible changes take place and what enormous meaning this will have in a person's life when these changes, due to disease, occur in the organism with ensuing disturbances of their function or injury to the whole.

Carriage

Carriage is the shapeliness and overall perfection of the entire build of the body. People with good carriages and correctly held bodies are pleasant to look at because they stand well and walk gracefully. It is also quite evident, that, thanks to a good carriage, all parts of the body are receiving normal nourishment.

The carriage of the human body is determined by the basic stem on which the whole body is supported, that is, the spinal column.

Medical science distinguishes between four types of carriages:

THE BASIC TYPE

Normal curves of the spinal column are well defined and have an even and undulating appearance. The vertical axis of the body begins in the centre of the skull, passes through the centre of the pelvic axis and in front of the knee joints. This is very much to the advantage of the human being. It is the ideal type of build. The elastic qualities of this type of carriage are the most perfectly adapted to handle harmful influences from outside such as lifting and bending.

THE FLAT TYPE

In the flat-backed type, the curves of the spinal column are slightly visible. The chest is flat and the stomach is pulled in. Firmness of the spinal column in this type of carriage is less. This type of column is easily damaged and is prone to sideways deviations.

THE ROUND TYPE

The round back resembles the basic type but has higher curves of the spinal column. The firmness of the column is high due to the round curves which give great protection to sideways influences which are caused perhaps by some types of violent involuntary movement.

THE STOOPED BACK TYPE

Here the dominating feature is the chest curve. This type may be placed between the basic and the round types of carriage already described.

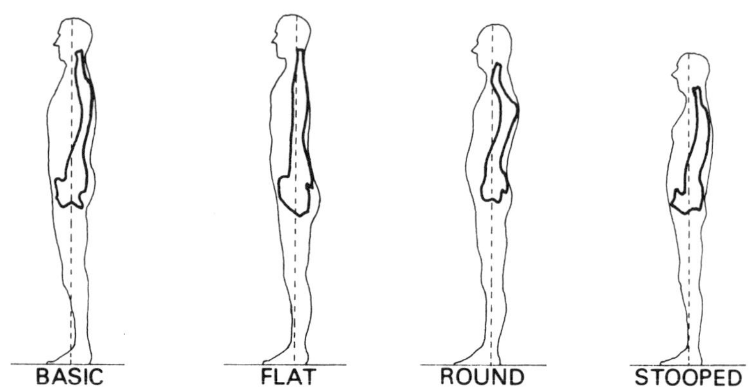

8. *The four types of carriage*

Of the four types of human carriage described, the most perfect type is the basic carriage, in which damage occurs only rarely, owing to the contour of its normal curves. Therefore the usual life sustaining processes of the human body can proceed normally.

The carriage of the body is the whole build of the human frame and its covering. People are born with one of these types of carriage but often a person's carriage is built and forms slowly during the life process.

It can be said that no other part of the human body reflects the social and professional way of life as much as the spinal column. A perfect carriage can be ruined through careless exercise or occupational stress. Likewise, a defective or poor carriage can often be improved or corrected by doing special exercises, by applying self discipline and even, in extreme cases, by changing one's occupation.

It will always be found that a person with a good carriage is one who breathes deeply and has strong abdominal muscles and that the muscles of the shoulder region and the back are also strong and of good tone. Such a person feels confident and bold. His movements are free and easy. Therefore it follows that the work capacity of such a person is very high indeed.

All the internal organs function correctly and actively. Impulses via the nerves, to all the organs, from the periphery to the brain and vice versa, function normally. Therefore, with a normal carriage, ideal conditions are created for a good blood supply, tone and assimilation and oxidation processes in the human body.

A careless attitude to one's body and consistently poor posture when walking or sitting not only weakens one's health but can make a figure look ugly. One is always immediately aware of a beautiful figure if it comes within one's range of vision and a well-controlled, smoothly walking body immediately attracts attention. Some people have the good fortune to be born with a perfect carriage. If that person is a woman and she uses her body to advantage, when walking, she will have that elusive and extraordinary grace desired by so many and given to so few. People with a correct carriage will not only look well but they will also rarely have suffering in their lower back. In other words, a correct, elastic, unconstricted and yet well-controlled carriage should be the goal of everyone.

Scoliosis

With the examination of the structure of the spinal column we saw that, regardless of its type, each spinal column has two forward and one rear curve which are normally formed during the first years of life.

Sometimes in a spinal column there is another curve, which normally does not occur. If it occurs it gives rise to a condition called scoliosis.

It is very important for everyone to know about scoliosis, particularly when there are children in the family. It is necessary to know why this curve occurs, how to prevent it happening, the treatment if it has already formed and the harmful effects it has on the body.

The word scoliosis comes from the Greek and Latin, *scolios* meaning crooked. Therefore in translation it means curved bones. Scoliosis is an abnormal curvature of the spinal column to either the right or the left side. Often it is accompanied by a dropped shoulder.

Scoliosis may be the result of one of a number of conditions such as poliomyelitis, rickets, traumas, malformation at birth, muscle fatigue and so on, but most often it is formed as a result of the harmful effects of an incorrect carriage or of certain types of work.

Depending on its origin, it is possible to distinguish many types of scoliosis but the most common are:

RHEUMATIC SCOLIOSIS

This is due to rheumatism of dorsal muscles.

SCIATIC SCOLIOSIS

Curvation of the spinal column toward the affected side in sciatica.

ISCHIATIC SCOLIOSIS

This type is due to hip disease.

INFLAMMATORY-OSTEOPATHIC SCOLIOSIS

Diseases of the vertebrae cause this.

PARALYTIC SCOLIOSIS

Lateral curvature of the spinal column.

LEFT-HANDERS' SCOLIOSIS

Very common in Australia.

HABIT SCOLIOSIS

Due to improper position of the body. Some very common bad habits are:

1. Writing at a low desk with one shoulder higher than the other.
2. Carrying a weight habitually on the same arm or shoulder.
3. Standing frequently with the weight on one leg.
4. Professional scoliosis (clerks, tailors, bootmakers, etc.).
5. School scoliosis.

SCHOOL SCOLIOSIS

One of the most common deformities of the spinal column is school scoliosis. Statistics given from many countries give a picture of from ten to fifteen percent of school children having, to a certain extent, symptoms of scoliosis. School scoliosis develops over a prolonged period of time and is the result of sitting in an immobile position for lengthy periods. Becoming tired from maintaining a strained vertical position, the child instinctively begins to hunch himself into a new position by bending sideways in either direction and resting the elbows on the table. This position becomes habitual and gradually the child develops scoliosis of the spinal column with all its complications.

Twelve or thirteen years, sometimes more, are spent by most young people sitting in school. It is not hard to understand what can happen to a child's spinal column, particularly in the chest region during this time, as an incorrect carriage develops.

The onus is on teachers to see that all students are comfortably seated. Because the students are in front of them daily for such long periods of time, teachers are in a position to note the habitually wrong and unhealthy positions in which a child sits.

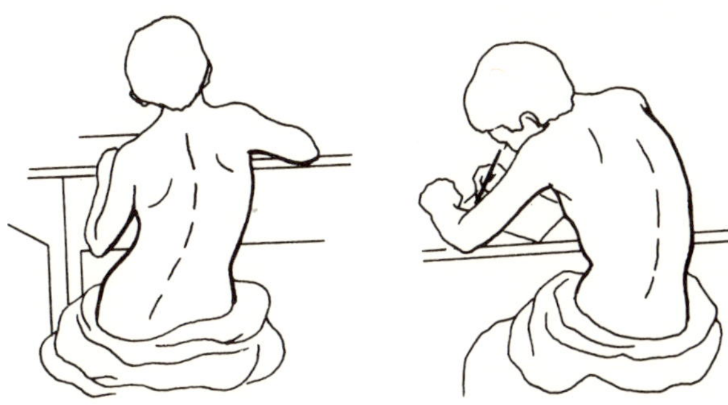

9. The types of school scoliosis

It must be realised that the development of this condition in the body can occur unnoticed with permanent and harmful consequences.

Scoliosis has particularly harmful effects on the functioning of the heart and lungs and on the lower regions of the spinal column.

WHAT IS INVOLVED IN THE PREVENTION AND TREATMENT OF SCOLIOSIS?

1. The maintenance of the correct carriage of each student during their years in school by daily exercises.

2. Massage and also physiotherapy.

In some cases, the wearing of a specially designed corset will help correct misplacements. Maintenance of a correct sitting position in the classroom or special corrective exercises also help.

Apart from insisting on correctly and comfortably constructed furniture for students (as far as it is within their power of course) teachers should monitor the carriage of each student. I feel that a short series of carefully selected exercises could be given to the children while sitting in their desks, at the beginning and end of each lesson.

The development of scoliosis during school life is increased also by an a-symmetrical load which children carry daily, such as an overloaded heavy school case, or bag, in one hand. It is a fact of nature that the right half of the body is heavier than the left and this leads so much more readily to scoliosis.

3. A third way to treat or avoid scoliosis is to rest by lying on the stomach.

4. Swimming on the back is strongly recommended.

5. Fresh air and sunlight are always beneficial.

6. Volley ball and basket ball are excellent corrective sports.

7. Take calcium and vitamins of Groups B and D, which strengthen bones and nerves.

CHAPTER 2

The mystery of the lower back

Of all the regions of the spinal column most often affected by disorders, the lumbar sacral region is the foremost.

It is not an exaggeration to say that seventy or eighty percent of all afflictions affect the lower part of the back.

It seems a contradiction of facts, almost a mystery, that the seemingly most strongly constructed part of the spinal column, consisting of only five of the largest and strongest bones and sitting firmly on the solid sacrum, should seem the weakest part and cause the most suffering, which often lasts almost the duration of one's life.

It is even more tragic that there is no guarantee that there can be a complete cure of the affliction and that it may return at any time, even for what seems an insignificant reason.

It is in this same region that everyone first experiences the alterations caused by degeneration of the cells causing pain which can be generally diagnosed as osteochondrosis.

The reasons for the weakness of this lower part are many and no one reason can be given as being more important than another nor can any be omitted since they are tied in with the structure of the human skeleton.

The first and basic reason for the weakness and frequent injury of the lower part is the lack of "shock absorbers" below the spinal column.

From the anatomy of the spinal column, we know that from the age of twenty-five to twenty-six, all the vertebrae of the sacrum and coccyx grow together into one large bone in which there are no discs. If these parts of the spinal column did not grow together, they would perform the role of shock absorbers or buffers, and would soften all the action in the lumbar region.

Take the Australian kangaroo, with its large elastic tail, as an example. This tail not only helps the animal to jump but also absorbs the shock of the jumps which can be of tremendous length and considerable height.

A human being has no tail. It probably disappeared many million years ago, when man gradually assumed a vertical position and the use of a tail as a shock absorber was no longer necessary.

The arches of the feet are the only remaining features which act as slight shock absorbers. People with flat feet are denied even this remaining absorber and therefore are more prone to injury of the lumbar region.

A second basic reason is that the discs and vertebrae which are located in the lumbar sacral region are the most active and overworked of the whole spinal column. Therefore, and quite naturally, they wear out at a faster rate than the others.

Thirdly, the lumbar region is the part which is most vulnerable and most often subjected to traumatic injury, especially due to falls.

Fourthly, the lower part of the spinal column carries the entire weight of the body and it follows, naturally, that the heavier a person is, the greater the pressure on the lower region.

Fifthly, the lower part is more prone to infection and chills.

Lastly, during pregnancy and childbirth, especially in a woman with a narrow pelvis, the lower part is greatly affected.

All these reasons give an insight into why the lower part of the back is so susceptible to the slightest injury.

CHAPTER 3

Afflictions of the lower part of the spinal column

During the past few decades disorders of the spinal column have increased to such an extent that they warrant serious consideration in industrial and medical circles.

According to European statistics, five percent of the population of Europe suffers with back complaints every year. What the percentage is in Great Britain can be judged by an alarming article written by Dr Matthews which appeared in a British medical journal.

"Backache costs more man hours than strikes. The problem is a huge one", Dr Matthews, a consultant at St Thomas' hospital in London, stated in a British medical journal. "Certified incapacity from back troubles in a recent twelve months' period was: 627 days in men and 347 days in women per thousand *insured,* and accounted for 33 percent respectively of all rheumatic complaints". He stated, "What is more startling is the time wasted compared to other reasons which grab the headlines more readily.

"Although these figures must be a gross under estimation of the total national figure, it represents over three times the amount of work lost through strikes," declared Dr Matthews.

In Australia, according to a Federal Government inquiry in 1977, two hundred and fifty thousand new patients turned to chiropractic treatment and possibly a third of the figure to medical doctors.

In the USA, chiropractors annually treat over one million spinal column sufferers. Again, this number does not include those sufferers who seek treatment from general practitioners and in hospitals. Even then, these figures do not give a full picture of the number of sufferers in any country, as a large number of people, especially those living away from the cities and towns, do not seek medical advice but endeavour to treat themselves.

In the opinion of Dr Henry Feffer, a famous orthopaedic professor of Washington University, the numbers of those suffering with spinal disorders are on the increase, especially those who have problems with the lumbar region (lower part), owing to an ever increasing sedentary lifestyle.

In this chapter only the most frequently occurring lumbar

region disorders will be discussed. Advice and instruction for more effective treatment will also be included as well as preventive measures. Because of the wide variety of ailments and medical treatments used I will limit myself to only a few of the more simple measures to be taken, particularly those I have used successfully during my many years of professional experience.

Inflammation of the roots of the spinal cord (radiculitis)

For the majority of people who have become accustomed to believing that all pains in the back are due either to a slipped disc, a pinched nerve or a torn muscle this new but correct name for pains in the back, will be confusing.

What is this pain?

What causes it and what is the treatment?

Let us talk about it and analyse it. It is important to know more about "cause and effect" because then the patient's pattern of living and the treatment of the disorder can be more effectively dealt with.

To further enlarge on the subject, I must diverge at this point.

Greek and Latin terminology are used in the practice of medicine. This tradition has existed for centuries, possibly even before the advent of the famous Greek medical genius, Hippocrates. Words such as vertebra, fracture, fibre and many others are quite common. But not as many people know that the word for bone in Latin is *os* and the ending of a word in *is* or *tis*, means inflammation. Sometimes two, and even three, Latin words are often combined to form one complex word. For example, osteo-arthritis consists of three words: *os*, *arthrite* and the ending *tis*. When combined, this means that arthritis has affected not only the joint but the bone as well. In contemporary medical schools, Latin is not learnt but in my student days all medical students were compelled to learn hundreds of Latin words and know them by heart for the examinations.

An interesting example of this is the word given to intervertebral discs which often cause people great discomfort. They have the incredible name of *fibrocartilagointervertebralis.* Thirty letters to make a single word! This name consists of five words joined together and brings to mind the happy word out of the Mary Poppins film, supercalifragilisticexpialidocious.

But let us return to this new name, radiculitis. The word *radix* in Latin means the root of the spinal cord and the ending, *tis*, means inflammation, hence radiculitis or inflammation of the roots of the spinal cord.

From the anatomy of the spine, we know that thirty-one pairs of spinal roots leave the spinal cord. These roots are the beginning of all the nerves of the human body. The roots of the spinal column and their covering are very sensitive to pain. They react very easily to every type of irritation or harmful influence (over exertion, tiredness, cold and injuries). Their reaction is expressed by inflammation, swelling, changing chemical reactions and pain. Disturbance of the blood and lymphatic circulatory systems occur, not only in the region where the actual spinal roots are found but in the surrounding tissue and often even further along the path of the nerves, which begin at these roots. All these conditions or factors together result in radiculitis.

Any part of the spinal column may be affected by radiculitis but most often it occurs in the lumbar region (lower back). My records show that from 75 percent to 80 percent of all spinal pain is found in the lumbar region. However. odd this may seem, the fact remains that the lumbar region is the weakest part of the spinal column.

With an inherited weakness in the spine, chronic chills, infections, heavy physical labour, over-straining and traumas, radiculitis may develop much sooner and affect quite young people.

Hundreds of thousands of patients with these symptoms turn to general practitioners. Even more go to chiropractors telling themselves that "something is out" and in many cases rough and unskilled handling increases the damage in the inflamed spinal roots, nerves, joints and the surrounding tissue.

During my long years of practice as a specialist of neurology and as a chiropractor, I have had hundreds of cases where the patients have told me that they could not stand rough manipulation. It made them feel worse. It increased their discomfort and often they could not move because of the pain and an ambulance would have to be called to transfer them to a hospital or back home. I regret having to admit that such things do happen. This type of manipulator will sometimes persuade the patient, at this stage, that he has three or five discs displaced.

All radiculitis conditions can be divided into two major groups:
1. Pain in the lower region of the back resulting from a chill, infection or arthritis. (This is simple radiculitis.)
2. Mechanical-physical damage of the lower part of the spine (traumatic radiculitis).

Simple radiculitis

There are three stages in simple radiculitis.
1. The first onset of pain responds easily to treatment and if the patient visits a doctor or physiotherapist immediately, the pain will disappear within three to seven days.
2. People who have a predisposition to radiculitis will take

longer to recover. It may be two or three weeks or even longer.

3. If the radiculitis does not respond easily to treatment, this usually means that the spinal column itself is already affected. Movement is difficult because of pain and weakness of the muscles. Pain is longstanding, persistent and extends to the groin or legs.

The stages described may not always fit precisely into these categories. There may be variations due to a different set of circumstances such as age, resistance of the body, response to treatment, and the actual cause of the disease. In most cases, however, it fits into the pattern described.

It is essential to remember that radiculitis tends to reoccur between periods of improvement ranging from a few months to a few years. People may feel they have completely recovered and then they do something which will bring back the condition. This usually happens with men, while at work, or perhaps it could be said that because of the type of work or situation in which they are most likely to be involved, men are more prone to reoccurrences of radiculitis.

Here is an example: a patient was a well-built, strong, physically fit man of forty-nine. He worked six or seven hours daily as a cutter in a meat factory and he had already had radiculitis twice. The first time was sixteen years previous to my seeing him and the second time only four years before. On both occasions I treated him with successful results.

He came to me a third time with an acute condition of radiculitis in its third stage. He had intense pain in the lumbar region of the back and in the right leg along the path of the sciatic nerve, so that when he walked he dragged his leg. The pain had been continuous for almost two weeks but he hadn't sought any treatment, thinking, or rather hoping, that the pain would finally subside. When I asked him what had happened this time to bring on the attack he explained that a widowed pensioner friend of theirs whom he had met at church had asked him to mow the lawn for her. He was half-way through the job when it started to rain but as he was anxious to finish the whole lawn he had kept going and finished up wet through. Next morning he could hardly get out of bed because of the pain.

What factors bring on radiculitis?

Medical statistics prove that in more than twenty-five percent of all radiculitis cases cold has been the cause. A chill or a draught may bring on a bout and it is interesting and important to note that a draught may be more dangerous than overall cold. When the body is exposed to overall cold, it mobilises all its defences to combat it, but a cold draught brings on a localised chill causing the roots of the spinal column to react with more severity and frequency.

Young people may often be seen speeding along on motor cycles with the lower part of the back exposed allowing it to be chilled by a continuous stream of cold air. These young people are definite future candidates for radiculitis and I have treated a number of patients whose problems began this way.

The second most common cause of radiculitis is infection and complications from other diseases (tonsillitis, inflammation of the middle ear, sinus, decaying teeth, infection of the ovaries, to name only a few).

There are particularly unpleasant forms of radiculitis caused by all types of arthritis. Arthritis is a degenerative disease of the joints and changes their form, so affecting the spinal roots. All these reasons account for a quarter of the factors causing radiculitis and back trouble.

Gout radiculitis is the name of what is commonly called just gout. Gout was always thought of as the disease of the old and the wealthy. (They enjoyed their liquor and could afford to indulge their tastes.) It was always thought to affect mainly the big toe, and supplied plenty of material for jokes and caricaturists. This is now known to be wrong. Gout may begin in any joint and affect people of any age. I have treated many young overweight people suffering from gout radiculitis in the spinal column. Gout appears when there is an increase of uric acid content in the blood which causes an accumulation of salt crystals in the joints. This leads to inflammation and pain in the joints and toffee-like thickening. There is also an accumulation of salt crystals in the discs of the spinal column, often in the chest area.

Gout is a chronic metabolic disease. Those who suffer from it are almost invariably large consumers of meat and alcohol and there is also often an accompanying lack of physical activity. In poor countries where the living standard is low, gout is almost non-existent. Unfortunately, in Australia, every fifth or sixth person, mainly males over forty-five or fifty, shows symptoms of gout arthritis which often affects the spinal column and causes elementary radiculitis.

Flat feet often lead to complaints of the lower back. This is a hazard affecting people who work in a standing position for long periods, for example, hairdressers, dentists and shop assistants. Of course there is the inherited flat foot factor as well.

Finally, a very common reason for the disease appears to be the disturbance of the normal position of the intervertebral discs because of the absence of blood circulation in the discs. Already at a relatively young age the discs begin to lose their elasticity and degenerate. As this happens, the discs are increasingly susceptible to injury.

A largely sedentary way of life and a tendency to be overweight usually go hand in hand with gout and radiculitis. Because of a lowering of the metabolism and the storage of fatty tissue, the blood circulation decreases, thereby increasing the accumulation of uric acid. Added to this, the base of the disc, the so-called fibrous ring, cannot withstand the weight of the body. The ring cracks making the displacement of the disc (slipped disc) almost inevitable. What follows of course, is that pressure is exerted on the roots of the spinal cord.

What type of person suffers most often with radiculitis?

Men suffer injury to the lumbar region of the back three times more often than women.

Paradoxically, when questioned, nearly every third or fourth woman over forty complains of having had a painful back for many years. In most cases these pains do not have a direct relationship to the spinal column. More often, they are muscle pains caused by housework or working in the garden, varicose veins, the menopause or as a result of some abnormality of the female organs.

But in any case, one must always bear in mind chronic continuous pain, as opposed to acute pain, in the lumbar region can be a sign that something is wrong with the female organs and it is both necessary and important to have a gynaecological examination.

It is important also, for elderly men who suffer with chronic lower back pains to have a prostate gland examination.

Children and young adults up to the age of sixteen rarely suffer pain in the lower back area except in cases of direct injury.

Freedom from back pain in the young is, without doubt, due to youth, mobility and good blood circulation in the spine. Their natural resistance to injury is much higher than that of adults.

Can radiculitis be hereditary?

Where radiculitis is the result of various conditions that have happened during the natural course of life (chills, arthritis, physical injury etc.), the tendency to the disease will not be passed on, of course. What is passed on is the constitutional make-up of the parents with their particular type (build) of spine. Inborn weaknesses and sometimes pathological defects, for example, spina bifida (the splitting of one of the shoots of the last spinal vertebra or the vertebra itself) can be passed on. Sometimes other very rare illnesses *are* passed on.

Is the number of spine sufferers increasing?

The answer to this question is, unfortunately, yes. There is a definite upsurge in sufferers owing to an increasingly sedentary way of life. Being sedentary affects us in the following manner. When a person is sitting down, pressure on the discs is twice as much as when they are in an upright position and this pressure is greatest in the lower part of the back. Therefore the increase is even greater for those suffering with lumbar region troubles.

Sooner or later everyone will suffer back pain. But the later it happens the better. It is simply a question of how long we can live before we have to fall a victim to a natural ageing process in which the body parts become less strong and more susceptible to pain.

Can radiculitis be cured?

To answer this question briefly is impossible. However, after fifty years of experience I can say that nearly half of all my patients have been completely cured. Most of these were in the young or middle-age brackets.

Again much depends on:

1. What stage they have reached.
2. The type of disorder.
3. The individual peculiarities of the organism.
4. Age.
5. Correct treatment from a qualified practitioner.
6. The common sense and self-discipline of the patient.

Naturally, those who take heed of the first "signals" of the disorder will recover more quickly and those who avoid excessive physical strain and exposure to cold are also better off.

To whom should you go to receive treatment for radiculitis?

Radiculitis must be treated by a qualified medical person. Don't be in a hurry and rush off for manipulation with the naive hope that one press or a twist to the spinal column, will cure you.

This is the most frequent mistake made by the majority of people, made because they hope for an "instant cure".

These people are often committed for months, even for years, to frequent visits to the manipulator, receiving repetitious manipulations which they really don't need. If these people had visited a physician in the first place and received correct medicinal and physiotherapy treatment they would have been cured at a very early stage.

The fault does not necessarily lie with the manipulator, but with the patient who is anxious for an early cure.

It should be clearly understood by everyone that you cannot expect the same expert treatment from a manipulator that would be given by a qualified doctor or physiotherapist. A manipulator will try to please the patients with standard and quick manipulation without proper analysis of the illness. Only a doctor can get to the root of the trouble and find out what is basically wrong with the spine.

CHAPTER 4

Mechanical-physical injury to the lower part of the spinal column (traumatic radiculitis)

Over fifty percent of injuries to the lower part of the back are the result of physical or mechanical causes which exert more pressure on the spinal column than it can resist. Over-strain occurs when weights which are very heavy are lifted without regard to the necessary weight lifting rules.

There are other types of injuries such as those caused by a fall from a horse, from a motor bike, from trees, roofs, and so on. Being stationary in a bent position for long periods has the same over-straining effect. Shearers, brick layers, carpet and lino layers, farmers and potato pickers, often suffer this type of overstrain.

Potato picking is a particularly hard and literally "back-breaking" job. It is really extremely wearing on the lower back.

Not many potato chip lovers realise how hard and "primitive" work is on some potato farms in Australia. It is necessary for the worker to bend, almost in a crouching position, dragging a bag between his legs, picking up the potatoes as he moves along the rows until it is half filled when at this stage the weight would be approximately thirty-one kilograms (seventy pounds). During this seasonal work the men are working from ten to twelve hours daily.

Certain sports contribute to the list as well. In football there is often hard physical contact which can be very dangerous. Often rodeo riders are prone to injuries that can lead to incurable paralysis of the limbs.

Injuries may occur after prolonged or sudden periods of vibration, particularly if the vibration is combined with a turning or twisting torso. Tractor and grader drivers as well as polocrosse players are victims of this type of hazard.

These examples are far from being complete with regard to the types of injuries that can happen to the lower part of the spine. They give but a brief picture of the whole spectrum.

There have been some extraordinary cases with which I have had to deal during my extensive experience. One was a farmer's son, a fine big fellow, and he and his brother astonished everyone with their weight-lifting capacities. He could carry on his back a bale of wool, weighing over one hundred and thirty-five kilos (three hundred pounds), three times round the house. However, one day while walking across a paddock, this Hercules stumbled slightly. The result was a displaced disc and a pinched nerve. For several days he was quite incapable of movement.

I can remember an almost fantastic case from the time, long ago, when I was a practising doctor in Germany. It happened on a building construction site. A piece of timber fell from a great height onto the head of one of the construction workers and it should have killed him. But the only thing that happened to this very lucky German worker was a fracture of the shoots of the last two lumbar vertebrae. He was able to return to his work a few months later. Of course complications from the concussion could have occurred at a later date but that has no relevance to our present subject.

All mechanical or physical injuries are combined into one large group called traumatic injuries. The word trauma means an injury which occurs from outside. The reader must keep in mind that all the traumatic injuries mentioned in the cases specified at the beginning of this chapter are included in this category.

Traumatic injury to the lumbar region of the spinal column disturbs the entire tissue structure of the human body. This can include skin, muscles, ligaments, tendons, blood vessels, nerves and bones.

Therefore it can be readily understood that injury will upset normal body functions and that the part of the body which sustains injury is particularly incapable of functioning correctly.

It is also easily understood that an injury affects not only the injured area but the whole body. If you have pain in your lower back then of course your nerves are affected. A person will sleep badly and may have a headache. The blood circulation in the legs may be affected and so bring on a feeling of pins and needles. The stomach and excretory systems may also be upset.

The reverse is also true. The general health of a person can have a tremendous effect on local pathological processes. A strong healthy body is more resistant to, and can more quickly recover from, local disorders. A weak or less resistant body will require more treatment and take longer to recover.

Injury in the lower region of the spinal column, as a result of trauma, may be of different kinds, and will depend on the degree of the trauma and on the condition or resistance of the spinal column of the person affected.

The most frequently occurring injuries to the lower back

1. Pinching or flattening of the roots of the spinal cord.
2. Damage to the muscles and tissue.
3. "Rupture" of the intervertebral discs (slipped disc).
   A flattened disc protrudes through the intervertebral opening. Nearly always the injured disc is between the fourth and fifth vertebrae in the lumbar region.
4. Spina bifida. A baby may be born with this condition.
   It is a split in the main (the largest posterior) outshoot of the vertebra and occurs in the lumbo-sacral region. From three percent to ten percent of the population is born with this abnormality. Spina bifida may be defined as "a variation of the structure of the lumbo-sacral region". The unlucky people born with this condition can often pinpoint the position in the sacral region where the pain is felt. Unfortunately, an X-ray will not always reveal this abnormality. Spina bifida appears at certain periods of one's life, usually as the result of physical strain.
   Russian orthopaedic observations have shown that the presence of an over-abundance of hair in the local sacral region indicates a greater than usual possibility of spina bifida posterior occurring. This hair phenomenon does not occur in women.

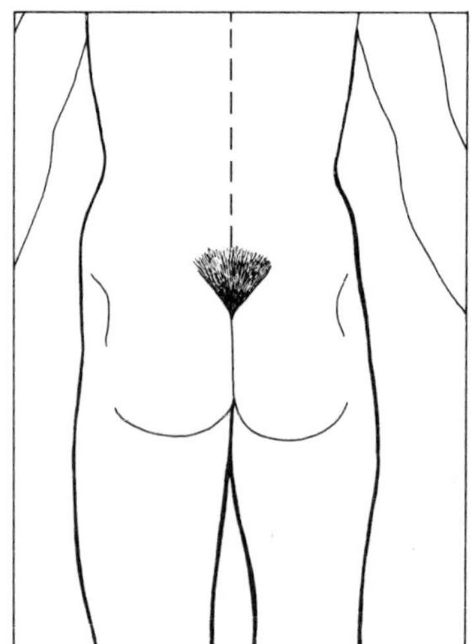

10. Over-abundance of hair in the local sacral region

5. Injury of the intervertebral joints (often between the fourth and fifth vertebrae or the last vertebrae of the lumbar and sacral regions.
6. Displacement of the vertebrae from normal positions (dislocation and subluxation).
7. Haemorrhage in the region of the injury.
8. Fractures of the vertebrae and their offshoots. This occurs only as the result of traumas of great force, perhaps a fall on the buttocks or back from a great height.
   There is also a large group of degenerative changes in the lumbar region which occur as the result of physical injury or because of various illnesses.
   Inherited abnormalities of the lumbar region may be present, causing it to malfunction.

The following conditions may occur as the result of injury to the lower spine:
1. Pain. Agonising pain the lower spine and often in the leg. The victim can neither bend down nor straighten up and may even collapse with the pain. The smallest movemet (a sneeze, a cough or a deep breath) will increase the intensity of the pain. In order to lift something from the floor it is necessary to squat without moving the spine. This pain occurs if the sensitive spinal roots are damaged or pinched.
2. Complete or partial paralysis of the legs.
3. Spasm. Contraction of the back muscles. These huge back muscles which lie above the injured region become subject to very strong contractions. Virtually, they bind the person as if with an iron hoop and lead on to the condition of left or right sided scoliosis (curvature of the spine to one side).
   The condition of the patient worsens to such an extent that any movement becomes impossible.

This state, a combination of agonising pain from the spinal roots and the contraction of the back muscles, is called lumbaco.

It also follows, and one should hear this in mind, that an attack of rheumatic lumbago may result from a chill. It affects only the back muscles, without scoliosis, and easily responds to anti-rheumatic treatment.

Of all the sections of the spinal column it is the lumbar region which succumbs most often to traumatic injuries, and it is mainly in the place where the lumbar and sacral vertebrae form the last joint. This is called the lumbo-sacral region. The name indicates that it involves both the lumbar and sacral sections of the spinal column with all their nerves. Traumatic radiculitis (lumbago) is not a frequent occurrence and happens mainly in cases of extreme injury. I would estimate that it happens in from five to eight cases in every hundred injuries. The majority of cases will be of average severity without the contractions of the back muscles.

Concerning women

It has already been stated that men suffer from traumatic radiculitis three times more often than women. This is logical because in Australia, the United States of America and in Western Europe, most hard physical labour is carried out by men.

But then the interesting question arises. Why is it that women in Asian and Communist countries, who share the hard physical labour with men, still have a lower percentage of traumatic injuries of the lower spine than men?

From my observations and having seen a very large number of X-rays of both men and women of approximately the same age, it is my firm belief that in women who have borne children, the intervertebral spaces in the lumbar region are considerably wider than in men. I strongly suspect that women have more flexible spinal columns than men. This greater elasticity gives women more protection in the spine so that it appears that women's physical design not only helps them with the physiological function of child-bearing, but it also gives them a spinal advantage.

During the period of pregnancy there is a gradual increase in pressure from the pelvis. This pressure affects the lumbar portion of the spinal column and so gradually widens the intervertebral spacings. It is a well-known fact that from about the middle of the pregnancy period onwards, the majority of women experience pain in the lumbar region of the back or at least have unpleasant feelings in that area.

The most sensitive parts of the female spinal column are the neck and thoracic regions between the shoulder blades. Here they most often suffer from chills of a rheumatic condition (fibrositis and radiculitis).

During my many years of practice, traumatic injury to the neck area of the spine was rare. There were two or three cases resulting from yoga exercises, mainly the head standing exercises, and all occurred in young girls.

A curious experience I must tell you about is of a physically strong farmer who brought his wife to me many times for treatment because of fibrositis and radiculitis of the neck. He insisted that a slipped disc in the necks of women occurred because they were "like cows — always wanting to look over neighbouring fences".

CHAPTER 5

Ground prepared

There is a period of "pre-condition" when the disease has not yet become active. However all the elements to activate the disease are there lying dormant and suddenly, often without warning, something happens and it is like a match applied to a petrol soaked rag — the conflagration erupts.

That may appear an over-dramatised description but is the most simple way of explaining what appears to be a sudden and inexplicable (to the sufferer) initial bout of illness.

It seems that the body is "ripe" for the condition to flare up and even an insignificant action may trigger it off.

An apparently healthy person is amazed to find that a crippling condition has appeared and to him there is no obvious reason why. The usual cry is, "I didn't do anything unusual. Why did it happen, doctor?"

This dormant condition only occurs in people who have previously suffered from pain in the lumbar region of the back.

There is an apt phrase in German which describes this unpleasant happening: *Hexen schus.* Roughly translated it means "witch's shot." In Russian, this happening is called a *prostrel,* or a "through shot" but the German phrase is more apt as it infers something demonic, only to be expected from a witch or a demon.

Occasionally, a perfectly normal, healthy person, may experience a temporary crippling condition brought on as the result of a slight movement, a deep breath, a cough or a sneeze.

The pain in the lumbar region may completely paralyse the person, making them cry out with pain. The victim clutches the nearest support, be it a chair or a person and is afraid to even attempt to shift as the slightest movement increases the agony. A person may become almost hysterical between crying with pain and laughing at his inability to move. A healthy person suddenly becomes an invalid. I have experienced this "witch's shot" twice myself. Let me relate one such happening.

The school holidays had ended and I was to take my eldest son to the city where he was to commence his university studies.

Everything was ready and I went to the bathroom to wash my hands.

It was winter and I could feel a chill coming on. I noticed the bath mat was not straight and went to straighten it with the toe of my right foot. Just an ordinary reflex action you would say. And there I was — immobilised, an agonising pain throbbing in the lumbar region which "paralysed" my legs and the whole of my body. My wife and son had to help me into bed where I stayed, completely helpless, for the next few days.

Another tragi-comic situation occurred with one of my patients. He was a retired farmer, sixty-seven years of age and had been suffering from spinal arthritis for many years. He was also an enthusiastic fisherman. (A hobby not recommended for arthritis sufferers.)

Once he sat under the town jetty, a favourite fishing haunt of the locals, until 11 p.m., shivering with cold and his feet dangling down towards the water. When he finally arrived home he warmed himself up with a hot cup of tea and a good tot of brandy and went happily to bed.

After breakfast next morning, as he felt fit and well again, he decided on another day's fishing. So when his wife went out to do the shopping he started to prepare his fishing gear. He felt the need to go to the toilet which was an outside one. While he was actually in the toilet he suddenly experienced agonising pains and he was forced to spend two and a half hours in this uncomfortable situation until his wife arrived home and helped him to bed.

These two examples illustrate quite clearly, I feel, that these sudden bouts of pain are not brought on by witches or evil spirits. In my own case, it was a chill. In my patient's case it was the prolonged exposure to the cold of the previous night, penetrating his entire body, that brought such disastrous results. The "ground had been prepared", the spinal roots were ready and waiting for these agonising pains to begin.

Many conditions can contribute towards this preparatory stage of affliction in the lower back. Most often it is over-exposure to cold (sitting for long periods on cold rocks or ground, long periods spent in wet clothes and cold winds or draughts). It can also be infections such as tonsillitis, 'flu, malaria and others. Periods of standing or sitting in uncomfortable positions are also provocative factors. Rheumatism and gout are also conditions that contribute to the preparatory stage.

Many of these conditions mentioned may not have any immediate after-effects on a physically healthy person but very often they prepare the way for a sudden attack of pain in the spinal roots of a person who has a record of suffering pain in the lumbar region of the spinal column. In such a person there is a weak spot — a place of weakened resistance.

Let us see what happens, and why, with the sudden onset of pain.

In these cases there can be no doubts about a slipped or displaced disc or vertebra as there was no physical action of the spinal column. Abnormal changes took place only in the actual spinal root and the surrounding cells. These changes involve inflammation and swelling of the spinal root and a disturbance of the blood and lymphatic circulatory systems (radiculitis).

Are there any symptons of the oncoming condition?

In most cases the person has an unusual feeling in the lumbar region and in the legs. There is a feeling — not quite an ache, not quite a pain, but there is a certain restlessness of the limbs and sometimes an awareness of coldness in the back. There may be that familiar tingling commonly called "pins and needles". However, these feelings are often ignored as the person knows he is a chronic back sufferer and attributes the feeling to a change in the weather or fatigue. He does not recognise them as symptoms of radiculitis.

What do you do when it happens?

In order to prevent an attack of agonising pain it is necessary to rest in bed. Apply some kind of gentle heat to warm the body, perhaps use an electric blanket or a well-insulated hot water bottle. A warm bath is very helpful. Take a dose of sodium salicylate, Dispirin or aspirin. *Under no circumstances have any manipulation done as any "adjustments" will increase the trauma of the inflamed and swollen areas.* Common sense and a little care should help the condition disappear and within two or three days, all symptoms will have gone and the chance of a relapse will be considerably lessened.

CHAPTER 6

The treatment of chronic disorders of the lower part of the spinal column

People suffer from chronic back disorders for a variety of reasons. Every elementary and traumatic back condition eventually develops into a chronic form.

In addition to this, if a person lives and/or works permanently in unhealthy conditions, then the chances of developing chronic radiculitis and arthritis are greatly increased. The climate may be damp or the working or living areas may have cement floors.

It was mentioned earlier that degenerative changes take place in the ligaments, cartilages and joints of the lumbar region of the spinal column as people grow older.

These changes have different names, according to their degree, the symptoms involved and the diagnosis. However, the diagnosis is still insufficient, although it helps to point the way to the correct treatment for the chronic radiculitis sufferer.

The treatment of chronic radiculitis may be carried out either in the home or at some outside location.

Home treatment

Home treatment may be successfully carried out particularly if the sufferer does not live alone and has someone to help him. The most important thing is that the person concerned must practise self-discipline and follow certain rules.

Home treatment consists of:
1. Treatment with medicine and vitamins.
2. Treatment with heat.
3. Treatment with movement.
4. Treatment with massage.

Let us talk about each of these methods.

Treatment by medicine

Treatment by medicine should only be carried out under a doctor's supervision and using his prescriptions. However, there are methods which do not include drugs and which do not have harmful side-effects on other organs of the body. In this group belongs the old and tested medicine sodium salicylate (pure or vitaminised). Also in this group are Ensalate, Entrosyalyl, aspirin and some others. Preparations in this group must be taken in fairly large doses but for short periods only (from one to a maximum of three weeks). There should be an interval twice as long between each course. The course should be repeated from three to four times, but once again should be supervised by a doctor.

In German this system of taking sodium salicylate is called *schtoss,* meaning a knock. It works more effectively than taking medicines for a prolonged period, perhaps for months or even for years. If medicines are taken over a long period they finally cease to have any effect, as an immunity develops. Added to this, they actually have harmful effects on other organs, particularly the stomach, liver and kidneys.

Treatment by vitamins

A very effective treatment for chronic radiculitis is the use of Vitamins B1 and B12. These vitamins are present in the different food groups but additional amounts of synthetic origin should also be included in the medicinal treatment. (Using synthetic vitamins is necessary because the amount found in food groups is insufficient for treatment.)

VITAMIN B1 (BETAMIN)

This is the most important vitamin for the treatment of radiculitis and is the one used for inflammation of the spinal cord and its roots and nerves. Apart from this, B1 strengthens and builds up the resistance of the whole nervous system against various harmful conditions.

B1 should be taken in large doses of from two hundred to four hundred milligrams per day, several times a year. The length of a course of Vitamin B1 should be from four to five weeks, with intervals of two and a half to three months.

VITAMIN B 12 (CYTACON 50)

This is an important vitamin, not only because it improves the blood quality but, and this is especially important, because it helps prevent osteoarthritis and inflammation of the peripheral nerves, particularly if it is taken in conjunction with Vitamin B1.

It is recommended that B12 should be taken in a dosage of one tablet twice a day in the same way as B1.

In many cases I recommend taking B1 and B12 on alternate days. In such cases the length of treatment by vitamins should be doubled. Instead of four to five weeks the vitamins should be taken for from eight to ten weeks.

It is important to know that Vitamin B12 is the only vitamin that contains metal (cobalt). With old age the metal content of the body grows less, and this vitamin can provide the needed metal for the body. B12 also activates the function of the liver.

An even more effective method of vitamin intake for chronic radiculitis is injection. The best result is obtained if the injection is made into the buttocks, but only into the upper outside quadrant, alternating between the left and right buttock. The injection form of Vitamin B1 is called Betasol. In extreme cases of radiculitis, Betasol Forte is recommended as it has a stronger effect. The injection form of Vitamin B12 is called Cytamen. Twelve or fifteen injections per course twice a year should be sufficient.

Treatment by injections does not necessarily have to be carried out by a doctor, sister or nurse. A member of the family or another person with experience in giving injections — even the patient — may give injections providing elementary hygienic precautions are taken.

Treatment by heat

Treatment of painful inflammatory conditions by heat has been used for a very long time. Sensible use of heat can have very beneficial results.

BATHS

I would place baths at the head of all treatment.

Salt baths are beneficial for people suffering with various forms of arthritis, radiculitis, diseases of the nerves and muscles. Also hot salt baths increase the loss of weight and so can be used beneficially by people who are overweight.

Ordinary bath water may be used but a better treatment is by mineral baths, which can be made by adding minerals if they are not already present in the water.

I believe firmly in treating inflammatory illnesses with mineral water. Many years of experience in spa resorts in different countries have shown me that mineral baths have very beneficial results.

I would strongly recommend home treatment by salt baths. Two double handfuls of stock salt, such as farmers use for animals, should be added to the hot bath. The best type of salt for use is that taken from "pink" lakes as it is rich in iodine.

Caution should be used when taking hot salt baths, as a bath of over forty degrees Celsius has a strong effect on the body. (See also my warnings about baths on page 41). Under the influence of hot baths there is a redistribution of blood in the body. The blood supply is increased in the surface, the skin, the muscles and the joints. The rate of metabolism is also increased. There is usually a large amount of perspiration and this facilitates the expulsion of the harmful substances which accumulate in the body. The heart beat is increased and the body temperature raised. In addition, if a mineral or solution is added, such as salt, mustard, or pine needle extract, then the effect of the bath is even stronger.

The length of time spent in the bath should be limited to fifteen minutes maximum. One should begin with a five to six minute bath and increase the time spent in it by only one minute on each subsequent occasion until the maximum time of fifteen minutes is reached. It is not essential or necessary to reach this fifteen minute maximum period. If, after eight or nine minutes you experience a feeling of lassitude, dizziness, a quickened heart beat or an unpleasant feeling in the heart area, you should immediately get out of the bath. Under no circumstances increase the time during subsequent baths, but, in fact, reduce it.

You should sit or half lie in the bath so that the hot water does not cover the left side of your chest which is of course, the heart area. Do not take a shower after a bath or the minerals will be washed off and it is much more beneficial to have the mineral residue left on the body.

During a hot bath and often after it, there is usually a large loss of fluid mainly due to perspiration. If the perspiration is excessive, then the loss of fluid should be replaced or dehydration may follow. A glass or two of water, milk, fruit juice or tea should be taken but under no circumstances drink alcohol.

As it is absolutely necessary to have a rest after a bath, it is a good idea to have the bath just before going to bed. Under no circumstances should a bath be taken after a meal or after the intake of alcohol. If the bath is taken during the day, it should be followed by a rest of one or two hours, then spend the next few hours inside, thus giving the body time to cool off and so lessen the chances of being chilled.

WHO CANNOT HAVE HOT BATHS?

You should never take a hot bath:
1. during pregnancy
2. if you have a temperature
3. when there are fresh or open wounds
4. if you have serious internal or blood diseases, such as high blood pressure, tuberculosis or suspected internal haemorrhages
5. if you are naturally very thin or weak.

The hot bath treatment should proceed gradually, beginning with one or two baths a week and if the treatment does not bring on any ill effects the baths may be increased to one each day. A course of treatment is from twelve to fifteen baths. There should be an interval of two or three months between courses.

Ray lamps and plasters

Both artificial and natural energy rays are utilised by plants, animals and of course, humans.

The application of heat rays for therapeutic purposes is

widespread, especially for chronic inflammatory conditions, nerve and muscle pain and muscle spasms. It is particularly beneficial for local application in radiculitis, especially when a patient cannot take hot salt baths.

There should be exposure to the rays from fifteen to thirty minutes preferably twice a day. Great care should be taken not to burn the patient. As with pain, especially intensive pain, the sensitivity of the skin is lowered and the patient is not aware of the penetrating rays and, in fact, often feels they are not hot enough.

Application of plasters also belongs in the domestic heat treatment method. There is a large variety of plasters that may be used but I would recommend the German mustard plaster, A.B.C. Its ingredients are active and have a prolonged effect and its use brings no complications afterwards.

Before applying the plaster, it is advisable to bathe the lumbar region with a wet, soapy flannel and then rub it with cotton wool soaked in methylated spirits. After which it should be dried thoroughly and the plaster tightly applied. It should be left on from twenty-four to forty-eight hours. After the plaster is removed, vaseline should then be smeared over the area.

In urgent cases, a good mustard plaster can be prepared in a few minutes in your own home. Dry mustard powder mixes easily with any kind of flour. Use a ratio of 1:2 or 2:2 (that is one part mustard to two parts flour, depending on the skin type, — for sensitive skins use less mustard). Slowly add hot, but not boiling, water and mix to a good consistency. Spread the mixture approximately six millimetres (about a quarter of an inch) thick over a cloth, place a similar cloth on top and the homemade mustard plaster is complete. Apply to the affected area of the body, cover the patient with a blanket or cushion or try to have him lying on his back so that the weight of his own body will add pressure to the plaster application.

From the moment the plaster is actually felt to be properly warm, leave it on for from ten to fifteen minutes, then remove it and wash with warm water.

Other beneficial home remedies include electric blankets, hot water bottles, warming the back with an iron through a blanket (ten to fifteen minutes), hot sand or salt (heated in the oven and put into a cloth bag) and hot foments (a towel put into hot water, squeezed out and applied several times to the back.)

With all these heat treatments, it is very important to bear in mind the skin type of the patient. The absence of pigment or a very white skin, is found especially in people with blond hair, or ginger hair and freckles. This skin is very sensitive to all types of heat treatment and burns easily. I have often seen patients with burns during my many years of clinical experience.

Ointments

With back pain, the rubbing in of pain relieving ointments is usually one of the first things people do when treating themselves at home.

Nearly all ointments, including those which contain bee and snake venom, have a salicylate base. That is the preparation I recommended in the section on medicinal treatment. In Australia a very widely used preparation is goanna oil. It compares favourably with other ointments and has more penetration.

However only normal and healthy skins should be subjected to the rubbing in of ointments. This should preferably be done after being warmed by a ray lamp, a bath or a hot foment because the heat opens the pores and allows better penetration of the ointment.

To cure radiculitis completely by the rubbing in of ointment is not possible, but regular and vigorous rubbing will be of great benefit and will help to relieve the condition. The effect of all ointments is twofold. The rhythmical massage increases the blood circulation and so improves the tone of the muscles, and the active ingredients in the ointments relieve pain.

Treatment by movement and massage

Because of their importance, treatment of radiculitis by these methods is explained in a special chapter of its own.

For self-massage of the lumbo-sacral region, an electric belt massage may be successfully used.

Treatment outside the home

This may be had in two ways:

PHYSIOTHERAPEUTIC TREATMENT

Which is possible only with a resident physiotherapist either in a hospital or in private practice. In most cases of radiculitis this is the basic form of treatment and combined with vitamin treatment and treatment by movement, gives the most successful results.

Under the guidance of a specialist physiotherapist, treatment may take the form of heat treatment, different electrical treatments, special exercises, or a short time of traction on a table or stairs etc.

HEALTH RESORTS

One kind of health resort treatment is balneological, which is treatment using mineral baths, spas and hot springs.

The basic therapeutic remedy is water from hot mineral springs which varies in chemical composition and temperature. This would be the oldest form of treatment in the world for all types of locomotor disorders, and also the most wonderful.

In the medical-therapeutic field its value was well known to both the Romans and the ancient Greeks. The hot sulphur springs were of special value.

Cribasius, physician in ordinary to the Roman emperor Julian, left precise instructions for making the best use of them. During the days of Imperial Rome, there were luxurious thermal establishments with beautiful surroundings. These were not only in Rome itself but were established by the Romans in all the countries they conquered including Britain, Germany and France. The Romans built bathing complexes including pools, which were surrounded by plants and gardens, columns and statues. Minerva, goddess of mineral waters, was always among their statues.

When Byzantine culture replaced the Roman, the use of mineral water and mud baths for therapeutic purposes continued to develop. Historical accounts of these practices, written in Latin, may still be found today in libraries in Rome and Genoa. Artistically illustrated, they show scenes set around sulphur springs where people received treatment and can be dated to a period between 1260 and 1275. The baths illustrated in these accounts were at Puteoli and Baiale in the Gulf of Naples. Unfortunately these baths were completely destroyed in 1538 by volcanic eruptions which were followed by an earthquake.

Now in many countries the treatment of all the organs of movement by the application of mineral water and mud, especially from hot sulphur springs, is widely used. For the treatment of chronic radiculitis, which in most cases has its origin in some form of arthritis, the most effective improvements are brought about by sulphur baths.

In my opinion the best of these baths are found in Rotorua in New Zealand. Due to continuous volcanic action, the water is rich in minerals which are important for the human body. Apart from this, volcanic mud is present in the water used for the baths: radioactive springs and sea water are also available. All of these ingredients make Rotorua waters most beneficial.

In some European countries bordering on an ocean there are bathing establishments near the shore into which sea water is pumped. The water is heated and people suffering from locomotor disorders have the benefit of hot sea baths all the year round.

A second type of health resort treatment uses mineral mud packs. Treatment by mud is one of the strongest and most effective of all forms of treatment. Whole body mud packs can be used by people with healthy internal organs. Local applications on only one limb or region may be taken by anybody without risk.

For therapeutic purposes, various forms of mud are used but all forms should be heated to a certain temperature before application. Mud may be silt, peat, mud from fresh or salt water, or volcanic lava.

For a course of treatment at a health spa, those fortunate enough may "live in" and receive balneological treatment.

Surgical treatment

Surgical treatment of the lumbar region of the spinal column (disc and other operations) should, in my opinion, only be a last resort action by the patient. During my long years of practice I have seen the results of many different types of operations and I cannot recall a single case in which the patient was completely cured and suffered no recurrence of pain. In quite a high percentage of cases, the condition of the patient deteriorated and they required further surgery which eventually led to a complete inability to work.

It is vital to remember that a patient who has undergone surgical treatment of the spinal column is already limited in regard to receiving other kinds of treatment.

To confirm my opinion I should like to quote the words of Henry Feffer*, a well-known American orthopaedic specialist who deals with problems of the spinal column. In answer to the question, "How risky is surgery on the spine?", he said:

> There is a risk. But the risk is more that the operation may not cure your back trouble, may even make it worse, than that you may die or be paralysed. You are much better off if you can get by without surgery unless your trouble is something very specific that only surgery can cure. Many patients should accept the fact that they are going to have some back aches and they should learn to live with them.

But of course there are some extraordinary cases when operative interference is vital. If the spine is fractured, if there is a tumour or there is a congenital defect, then only the surgeon's skill can begin to help.

MINOR SURGERY

In this category is included surgery which is not directly related to the spinal column itself. Such surgery is not dangerous to the patients. It will not cripple them or endanger their lives, in fact the results may be highly successful.

Sometimes it is necessary to perform a lumbar puncture. This is the injection of an analgesic substance into the spinal canal. Analgesic substances can be injected without a lumbar puncture. There are also substances which can be injected into the disc itself in order to make it contract, thereby reducing its protrusion.

*"All About Back ache", An interview with Dr Henry Feffer, *The Reader's Digest,* June 1972.

During the last few years, some doctors have made a practice of cutting the nerve in the region where the patient is suffering the pain. This system is called rhizolysis and sometimes it gives positive results. Very fine surgical instruments are inserted to a certain depth into several places along the path of the spinal column and the doctor, with certain movements, attempts to cut the nerves which project from the spinal column. The negative effect of this method is that the doctor operating cannot see what he is doing and I call this "a blind operation". Personally I am not in favour of these surgical attempts on such an important and delicate part of the body as the spinal column and I would not take the responsibility of recommending this method of treatment to anyone.

CHAPTER 7

Treatment of traumatic injury of the lower part of the spine

Treatment of injury of the spinal column, particularly the first time and if the injury is the result of a trauma, calls for caution, experience and definite medical knowledge.

Standard treatment of these cases, without a preliminary medical examination and an analysis of the nature of the injury, is always risky and may sometimes lead to irreparable harm. *For this reason, it is better to receive no treatment at all than treatment from an unqualified person.*

First aid

With mechanical-physical injury in the lower region where there is severe pain, even if there is no suspicion of a fracture, I would never recommend immediate transportation of a patient. Always remember that transportation, particularly over a distance and in an uncomfortable position, (there are not always facilities for transporting a person in a lying down position) may do him more harm than good.

The most important thing is to keep calm and not to panic. Try to get the patient into bed and he will then find the most comfortable position himself for his body. Do not complicate the issue and cause the patient unnecessary pain by attempting to put boards under him or place him on the floor. Put a low pillow under his head and a small one under his knees.

Warmth is not recommended with severe pain, because it can often increase pain. In many cases, pain is relieved by local "freezing". Place a plastic bag filled with ice on the lower region. Temporary freezing of the injured area with Skefron, according to the instructions, is even more effective for the rapid relief of pain. It is a good idea to always keep Skefron in the house, particularly if you live away from towns.

Perhaps two or three times a day the patient could be given aspirin, Dispirin or Panadol, depending on what is available. It is best to abstain from alcohol.

In a day or so, when the pain has lessened, heat treatment with a ray lamp may be used combined with light massage and the gentle rubbing in of an ointment. This could be done after a bath and in the evening just before going to sleep.

It is better to wait until the worst pain subsides before taking the patient to a chiropractor or a hospital for treatment. Apart from the harm that may be done by immediate transportation or shifting of the patient, any treatment given will be of little or no benefit because he is in an acute stage of lumbago.

Treatment in the hospital

Only serious cases which warrant special care and observation need hospital treatment.

Treatment in a hospital has certain advantages. Firstly, patients are completely away from the temptation to do any domestic chores. They are, to an extent, barred from any physical exertion and therefore receive the complete rest which is of such vital importance, especially during the first few days after the injury has occurred.

Secondly, patients are under constant medical observation and will have thorough medical checks. The third advantage to hospital treatment is that medical advice and help are directly available to the patient and the question of transportation does not arise.

There are disadvantages too, however. In most hospitals, chiropractic treatment is not available and some patients with injuries of the spinal column need it. Most general practitioners are not only sceptical about its benefits but actually have a negative attitude towards it. Therefore chiropractors in hospitals are rare.

As a doctor myself I fully understand the unfortunate circumstances that have made this attitude so common.

Chiropractic treatment

WHAT IS CHIROPRACTIC TREATMENT?

The modern American Medical Dictionary describes "chiropraxis" as "a system of treating diseases by manipulation of the spinal column" and a chiropractor as, "one who practises chiropraxis".

Chiropraxis is quite young in comparison with such treatments as acupuncture, hydrotherapy, homeopatherapy, osteotherapy and physiotherapy: it is only about seventy to seventy-five years old. Bearing in mind the short time it has been practised and the opposition to it from contemporary scientific and medical establishments, chiropraxis has become very popular in a comparatively short time and has received official recognition in many countries. Without exaggeration, it may be said that several million people go through this form of treatment every year in the

USA, Australia, Canada, New Zealand and other, mainly English speaking, countries.

Of course it is very difficult to say what percentage of patients are completely cured, what percentage receive only temporary relief, how many receive no benefit from it at all and how many are actually made worse or whose conditions are complicated and worsened by chiropractic manipulation. No one can answer these questions honestly and accurately. Unlike standard medical science, chiropraxis does not have statistical records. Apart from this no clinical or pathological observations are on the whole, possible.

Why then is chiropraxis so popular? Perhaps it can be explained by the following:

1. Chiropraxis offers a quick cure so it is understandable that so many people want to try it.

2. From a purely psychological viewpoint, any new system or method is always popular when it is introduced and there is even a saying that "one must hurry to be treated by new methods and systems".

3. The most important aspect of chiropraxis when it is judged or looked at impartially, is that the results are often successful where ordinary medical help has failed. In some cases, pain in the lower region may be reduced by a chiropractor when a general practitioner's treatment was insufficient or unsatisfactory.

If it can be said that only two or three out of every one hundred people suffering with pain in the lower region think that chiropractic treatment has either helped them or cured them, that alone is a good advertisement for it. These two or three successes (forgetting all about the failures) are enough to ensure the popularity of this method of treatment.

Those people who perform spinal column manipulations often refer to D.D. Palmer, an American who talked on this subject with authority during the latter part of the nineteenth century. He maintained that he had discovered a method of spinal adjustment and further, that all diseases were due to subluxation of the vertebrae and could be eradicated by adjustment of the vertebrae. Palmer died in 1912 without having explained to anyone the origin of his idea for spinal adjustment, but he had many followers to continue his theories.

Palmer claimed to have cured by his method a patient who had been deaf for seventeen years. At our present level of medical science such a statement sounds more like a fairy story than a solid fact. Palmer couldn't have known what we now know: that the eighth pair of cranial nerves, the auditory nerves (or the nerves with which we hear) have no connection with the spinal column at all. Fibres of the hearing nerve begin in the middle ear which is found in the temporal bone of the skull. The hearing centre is found in the crust of the temporal part of the brain. Even if we stretched reason to almost impossible lengths and, by hypothesis, said that the hearing nerve was being pinched (which is completely impossible) it would still be a fact that no nerve can be restored to its normal functioning action after seventeen years!

Occasionally there are cases of nervous-hysterical muteness and paralysis. These are rare and occur as the result of shock. They can be cured, but usually only by shock treatment.

Palmer's theory about treatment was based on unstable foundations, but he did confirm that subluxation and dislocation of the vertebrae (that is their displacement) are root causes of many illnesses. Contemporary chiropraxis is now mainly based on the displacement of the intervertebral discs which is much closer to the facts of current medical science.

Unfortunately, Palmer's most important point has yet to be confirmed. It is that the methods of chiropraxis may treat and cure most illnesses. Therefore it is understandable that there is, from medical practitioners, both criticism and a negative response to the whole system of chiropraxis.

Let me list those illnesses which the American Research Foundation and some chiropractors claim can be treated.

Appendicitis	Disease of the eyes
Diabetes	Pneumonia
Epilepsy	Disease of the thyroid gland
Haemorrhoids	Disease of the bladder
Parkinson's Disease	Rheumatic Fever
Diseases of the kidneys	Disease of the ovaries
Yellow Fever	Menstrual disorders
Angina Pectoris	Skin diseases
Heart disease	Even running noses

Reading this, a person with any intelligence might smile in disbelief. However there is still a grain of truth in it or perhaps one could say, at least "a healthy kernel".

Chiropractic treatment consists of fairly plain, standard, manipulation of different parts of the spinal column. These are called "adjustments" which open the joints of the spinal column by means of quick, rough movements of the spine.

Approximately fifty to sixty percent of patients having this type of treatment suffer severe pain and great discomfort. In many cases, the opening of the joints brings the patient temporary relief from pain and sometimes there is a complete "magical" cure.

The opening of the joints forcefully releases the spinal roots from pinching. The portion of the disc that is protruding, like a hernia, may slip back into the intervertebral space, giving the patient relief from pain within a few minutes.

I must repeat that in many cases of traumatic displacement, manipulation of the spinal column can be very successful and I have proved this repeatedly with my own patients.

In London's St Thomas' Hospital, the Honorary Consultant in Orthopaedic Medicine, Dr James Cyriax,* a leader in his field, uses spinal manipulation with great success for many of his patients. Judging from the illustrations in his excellent book his manipulations are identical to those used in chiropraxis. Dr Cyriax recommends those manipulations to physiotherapists and general practitioners.

What is of concern with the displacement of vertebrae (subluxation and dislocation) is that these injuries are much more serious than most people realise but they do not occur so frequently and are usually the result of severe injury. Displacement of the vertebrae happens most often in the mobile parts of the spinal column, that is the neck and the lumbar region. Dislocation in the neck is particularly dangerous. It is well known that if the correction of subluxation and dislocation is not done by an orthopaedic surgeon, paralysis and death can follow.

Treatment of dislocation must be done under a general anaesthetic and followed by a complete rest in bed for a few days. Under no circumstances must this manipulation be attempted in a chiropractor's surgery.

Manipulation on the joints of the human body, particularly after hot or steam baths, was known even in the ancient worlds of Greece and Rome, and was carried out by specially trained slaves.

In Turkey, Old Russia and other countries, mainly Asian, there was, and still is, a special person in the public baths who, for a small extra charge, will do manipulations for clients. When I was living in the Caucasus and frequenting the public baths, I often saw a thin Tartar, with only a towel round his waist, treating people for various conditions. After they had taken a hot or a steam bath, he twisted the joints, then, carefully walking over his client's back, would pause for a time in a certain place, concentrate, and, then suddenly would press down with his heel, causing a click.

Perhaps D.D. Palmer was once a client in a Turkish bath house and got his adjustment ideas from there. Maybe! In any case, not the Turkish Ali Bàba or the Russian Ivan, but D.D. Palmer

---

* James Cyriax, *Textbook of Orthopaedic Medicine Treatment by Manipulation, Massage and Injection (published in 1976)*

"enriched" American medical science with his method of adjustment and called it chiropraxis.

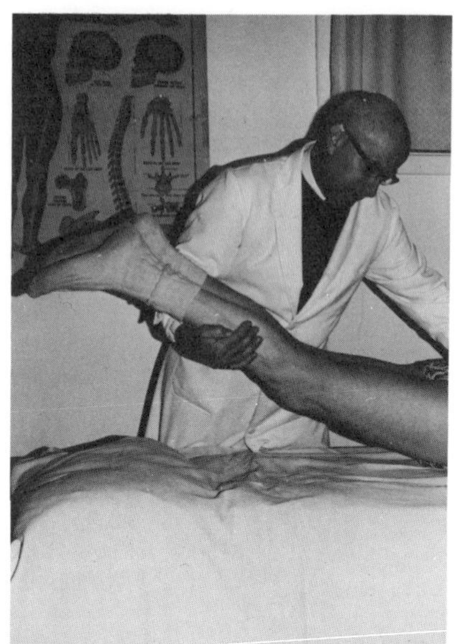 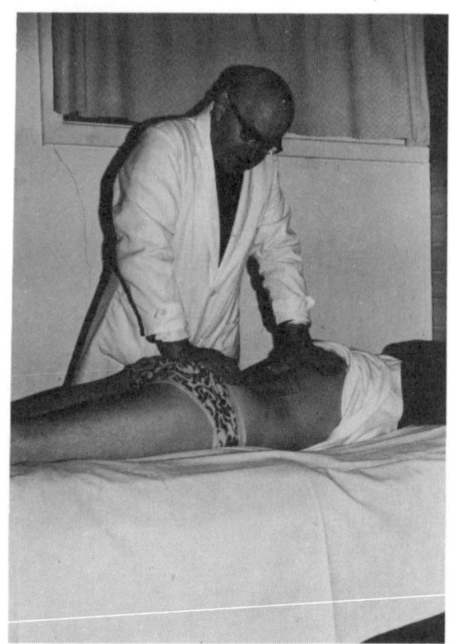

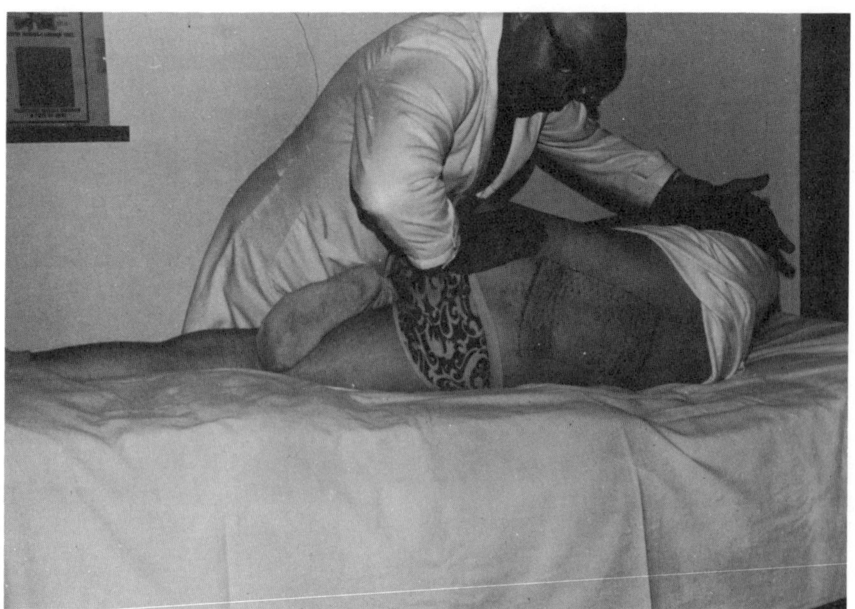

11-13. *Standard chiropractic manipulations for lower parts of spinal column*

CHAPTER 8

X-rays

In 1895 a German physicist named Roentgen discovered rays invisible to the human eye which he called X-rays. These rays pass easily through various kinds of dense matter including the human body.

X-rays are used widely in science and technology, but first and foremost their greatest use is in the field of medicine. They are harmful if used indiscriminately. Precautionary measures must always be taken when they are being used and those people working with them must have a thorough and skilled knowledge.

An X-ray of a normal spinal column will show quite clearly the contours of the vertebrae and the free spaces between them. Discs and spinal roots will not show up on an X-ray.

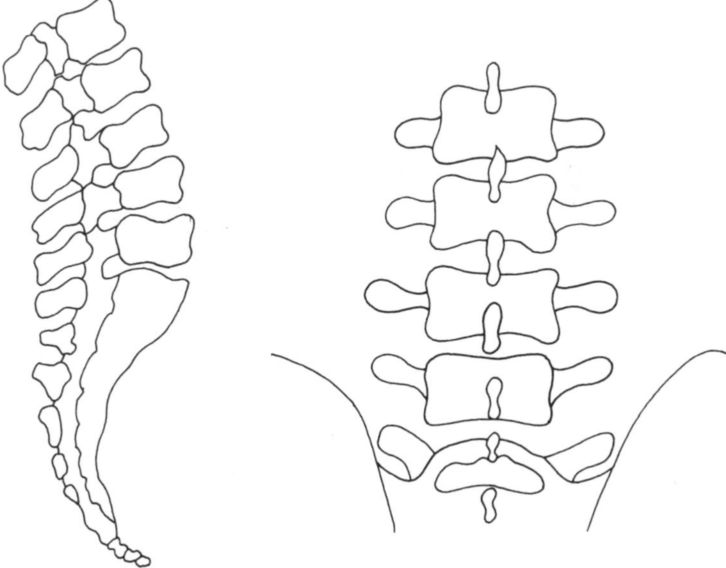

14. *Normal lumbar-sacrum and coccyx (lateral view)*

15. *Normal lumbar region from the front*

X-rays of the lower spinal column are very useful in revealing what state it is in and to see if any pathological changes have taken place, such as curvature, fractures, cracks, displacement, shrinkage of intervertebral spaces, calcification of discs, genetic defects, and so on.

People who suffer with recurring disorders of the lumbo-sacral region would be well advised to have X-rays taken every three or four years as these periodical observations could prove a preventative measure against the condition deteriorating.

It must be remembered that X-rays are not a treatment but a way of helping the practitioner to establish the condition of the spine. How useful and important X-rays are in diagnosis can be seen in the following illustrations which show various changes in the spinal column.

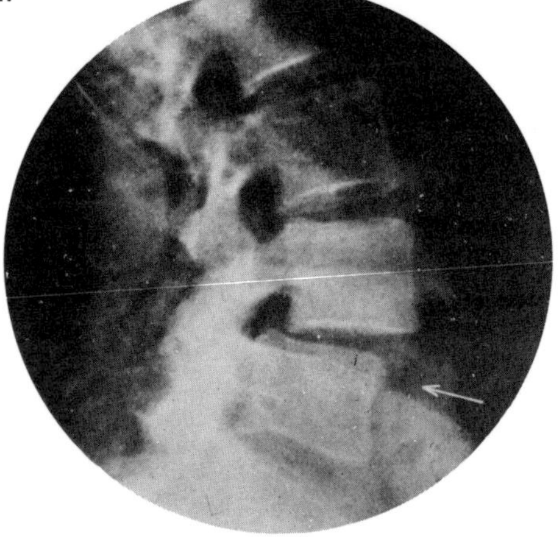

16. Dislocation of third lumbar vertebra

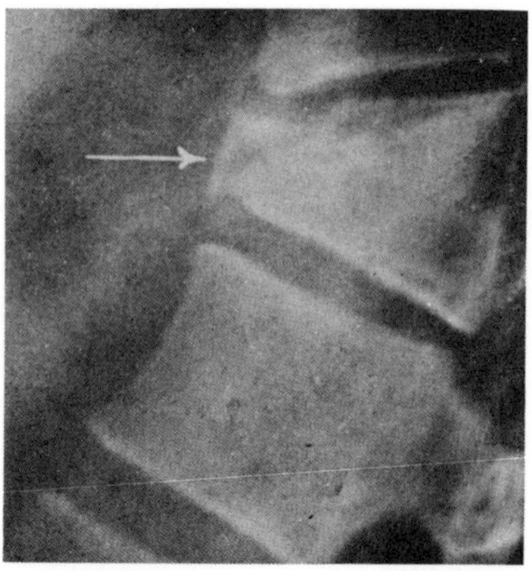

17. Worn out lumbar vertebra

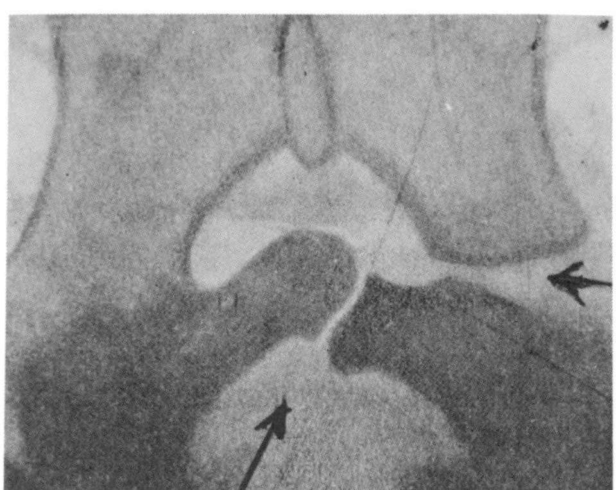

18. Double split (spina bifida)
of the fourth lumbar vertebra

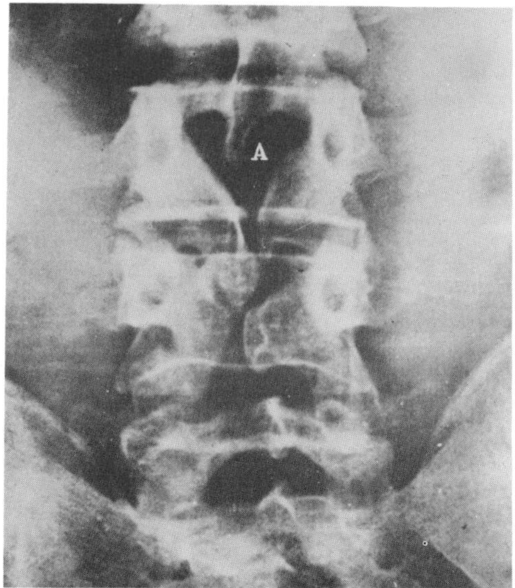

19. Spina bifida of the second,
third and fifth lumbar vertebrae

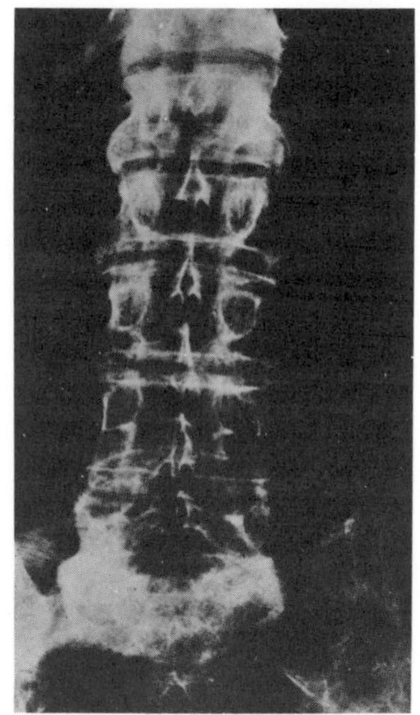

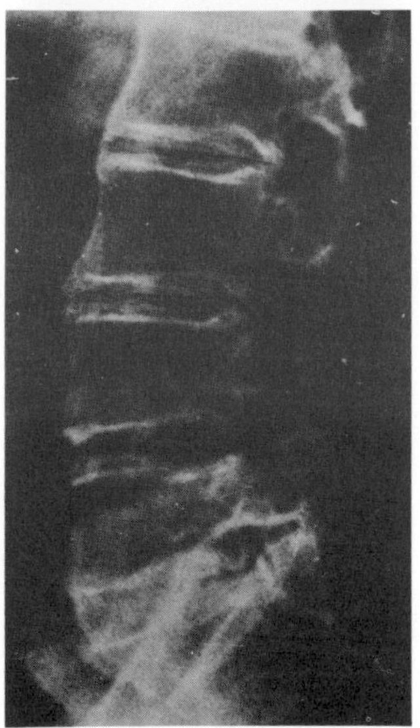

20-21: Typical pictures of
arthritic conditions of the lumbar
vertebrae with calcification of
intervertebral cartilage

CHAPTER 9

Treatment by movement

During the course of the last decade, our bodily activities have lessened to an alarming degree. Heart disease and disorders of the lungs, blood vessels and organs of movement, including the spinal column, have become sufficiently common to cause alarm in the medical world.

There is no doubt that the modern lifestyle is the main cause of sickness in the twentieth century. Television, motor bikes, cars, buses, trains and planes, not to mention noise, radiation and pollution, increase the likelihood of disease and shorten the span of human life.

The inadequacy of human movement may have once been compensated for by exercises in the form of sport and games in the fresh air. But this is offset now by the very real problem that modern man has little time for these activities. Added to this factor is the special problem of middle-aged people. Sport is mainly for the young, the healthy and the early middle-aged groups. These include the people who take part in team events and competitions. Sport for the masses is practically non-existent and the majority of people are merely passive spectators or "take their sport" sitting in front of television. For this reason, the one solution to the problem may be in individual gymnastic exercises which must be performed by each person until old age or infirmity bring them to an end.

Life is movement. *Without movement there is no life,* says an old Greek proverb. Or in other words, we can walk as long as our legs will move but to keep our legs moving, we must walk.

Treatment of the lower portion of the spinal column by activity is so important and so vital that, without doubt, I should place it second in importance to manipulation, although special exercises and certain types of games and sport may be of definite advantage and will have positive effects only if they are approached with a serious attitude and are carried out according to the following instructions:

    1. they must be carried out regularly and thoroughly

2. they should not be performed jerkily or in a rough manner
3. they should not be lengthy or tiring
4. they must cease at the first sign of pain.

Walking

The basic and most important form of exercise is walking. All physical exercise should begin and end with walking and it should be part of one's life up to and including, old age.

Walking prepares the heart for all types of physical strain and also gradually calms it down afterwards. Walking has an advantageous effect on health. It calms the nervous system, aids the work of the heart and lungs, strengthens the muscles and raises the rate of metabolism.

If commenced systematically, as a form of exercise, the first walks should be from twenty-five to thirty minutes long. They should gradually be lengthened to two one-hourly periods daily. One should take one walk in the morning and the other in the evening, preferably after the evening meal.

With chronic, as opposed to acute, disease of the lumbo-sacral region the best exercise is walking, but never running.

From the age of forty or forty-five, gradual and hardly noticeable changes begin to take place in the bone and joint formations of the system, including the backbone. Those people who do little or no walking begin to feel the effects of old age creeping on especially in the legs and in the lower back.

Walking should be done frequently. Inclement weather need not be a deterrent as walking can be done indoors, either on the spot or around the house. There are different types of walking; you may stroll slowly, march briskly or walk on the spot. One must choose the type of walk to suit the condition of one's back. Age is a major consideration, as is also the ability to move, whether or not pain is felt, and the length of time between urination. Therefore you should decide for yourself on the types of walking you will undertake.

The most important point which deserves mention is the correct position of the spinal column while walking. The spine-torso must always be kept straight. The shoulders should be held a little back and the head raised high. When walking, swing the arms a little and occasionally place them behind the back and then on the hips. Try to walk in one straight line.

It is especially important for women that they do not swing the hips.

Correct breathing is vital. The size of the step will be

governed by the length of the leg and one breath should be taken every three or four steps. It is better to walk alone or in companionable silence with someone, as talking breaks the rhythm of breathing.

Correct footwear is of great importance. It should be comfortable, and light; perhaps some type of sports shoe, as very high heeled shoes cripple the feet.

Swimming

Swimming would rate second only to walking as an exercise and is extremely important in the treatment of most physical injuries.

In the case of injury of the lower portion of the spine, swimming is most beneficial if carried out after a walk and then a short rest.

Walk into the water gradually. Do not run and dive in.

Swimming on the back is recommended in preference to other styles. Move the legs into a squatting position like a frog (i.e. like an inverted breast stroke leg movement) and then stretch them out straight.

For those who cannot swim, sea bathing is still advisable. Wade out until you are waist deep and keep moving around. Don't stand still like a telegraph pole!

Under no circumstances remain in wet bathers after the swim or allow them to dry on your body. Change as soon as possible. Avoid cold winds and rest in a comfortable position for half an hour or an hour but *not* on cold wet sand. If you can find dry hot sand on the beach, bury yourself in it.

Treatment by swimming is only sensible in warm, dry weather. It is well to remember that year-round swimming is not beneficial to everyone and that only completely healthy and "tough" individuals can attempt such a rigorous course.

Golf

Of all the types of games, golf is the most perfect one from a medical and psychological point of view, although some people may question the validity of the second part of that statement!

Due to the smoothness of the correct movements in this game and their variety (walking, bending, twisting) and the fresh air and usually delightful surroundings in which it is played, golf benefits not only all parts of the human body, but the mind as well.

From the point of view of treatment, golf can be recommended to people of all ages. It not only helps to correct physical defects but also helps with the treatment of the nervous system.

During thirty years of chiropractic experience in my home town, which has four golf courses, I have never had to treat a case of lumbar injury which resulted from playing golf.

Golf is not only possible, but highly recommended, for those suffering with their spinal column. If you are a golfer, play more often but not more than six to nine holes. Walk calmly around the course, don't strain the muscles by attempting to hit the ball too hard and too far and always remember that you are playing for treatment and exercise but not for records.

Special exercises

Even today there are many people who still think that exercise should only be practised by the young and physically fit. This idea is not only erroneous, it is harmful.

Exercise should be undertaken by everyone including pregnant women and convalescing post-operative patients. It is of special importance to exercise in old age and if one is suffering with back complaints.

What happens is that, with age, the muscles and tendons shrink, the flexibility and movement of the joints decrease and joints become drier because of the accumulation of minute crystals of different salts, and the disappearance of the lubricating fluid. Because of these factors, movements become slower, tighter and often painful.

People who suffer with painful joint movements think they should move less or perhaps it would be a more valid statement to say that they prefer to be less active. They sit or lie down more often. This results inevitably in a gain in weight and a deterioration of their condition. They go from one doctor to another, try one remedy after the other, listen to many willing and unprofessional advice-givers, unaware that the best and simplest remedy for many illnesses is to get off their chairs and move their bodies.

There are countless systems and methods of exercise which I won't attempt to analyse at this point. Each system has some merit and it is clear that all systems have some uses and advantages to the lower region of the back. It is necessary to find out which method suits *you*. The choice of the right movements for you is of vital importance. Often patients themselves feel that they need exercise. They see how football players train and think that this type of exercise will be good for them as well. But instead of doing them good it will probably prove disastrous.

For treatment of the lower region of the spine I recommend the following four simple exercises which have proved highly successful in my experience. They must be done regularly but never during bouts of acute pain.

The first three exercises should be done every morning, preferably in bed. But they may be done on the floor on a comfortable mat or rug.

1. Place the hands firmly on the hips and slowly raise each leg in turn without bending it. Repeat five times to begin with and gradually increase during the following days until you are exercising each leg fifteen times.

2. Bend the legs at the knees, place hands on knees and force the legs apart, then bring them together again. Begin by doing this ten times daily, gradually increasing to thirty times at each session.

3. Lie on your back, raise your arms above your head and take a deep breath, stretching your body to its fullest possible extent. Repeat this three to five times.

4. This exercise, consisting of four movements, is illustrated in figure 22. It should be done in a standing position. Stand up straight, spread the legs apart and raise the arms to just above shoulder height on each side as in Step 1. Without lowering your arms, slowly turn the torso (body) first in one direction and then the other until it will go no further, as in Steps 2 and 3. After these two movements, without lowering the arms, slowly bend sideways as far as possible, just one side and then the other, as in Steps 4 and 5. Make certain that your arms are in a straight line during the entire movement, and that you stretch your arms at the same time. Remember, this exercise consists of twelve movements, six twisting *and* six sideways bends.

Exercise is most important because it opens all the joints of the spinal column. If these exercises can be performed without provoking a bout of pain, then after a few weeks, they should be done twice a day. Never hold your breath while doing them but breathe freely and naturally. Do not do these exercises before going to bed or too soon after a meal.

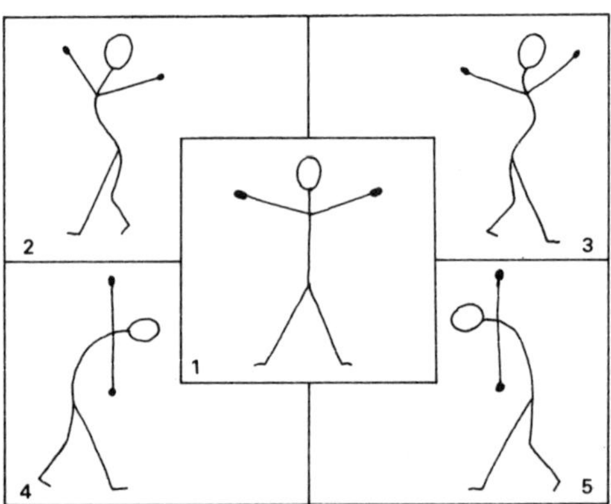

22.

I do not recommend other exercises involving the lumbar region, especially those involved with touching the toes without bending the legs or bending backwards using a wall support. These bending exercises are meant for healthy people free of back trouble.

To conclude this section on treatment by movement, I must again remind readers that treatment by movement must be thought about seriously, and carefully, and not rushed into without proper consideration. Remember that movement is treatment, but not every type of movement is beneficial and some may even be harmful and *could* result in damaging side-effects.

During my life there have been many times during surgery hours when I have suggested the necessity for exercise to a patient, only to receive the somewhat tart rejoinder, "Thank you doctor but I already get plenty of exercise at work." When this happens I reinforce my advice by actually demonstrating the exercises myself. I also show the patient what occurs in the spinal column by using a model I have and emphasising the point with the use of X-rays.

I also tell them, "If you chopped wood every day for half an hour, this would give you exercise, but if you chop wood every day for several hours then this isn't exercise but hard physical labour. The latter will have a harmful effect on certain parts of your body and to correct these affected areas, other physical exercises will be necessary."

As an example, shearers, bricklayers and men who lay carpet all work in a bent position and they all need special exercises to straighten the spinal column. They need the joints opened which have been closed during their work. I'm glad to say that most of my patients seem to understand what I am trying to convey.

In conclusion I must give a warning. People who have lower back pain and disabilities should not take up any sport involving sudden or jerky movements. Football, soccer, squash, tennis, cricket and badminton are all examples of this type of movement. Sudden or jerky movements can easily provoke more trouble. And I must also warn against games which involve bending the spinal column in one direction only and then standing still for considerable periods of time. Lawn bowls is an example of this type of game.

Gardening

It is necessary to say a few words for those people who enjoy gardening. There is no question about it being not only a healthy form of exercise but also a pleasurable hobby. Working quietly in the fresh air amongst flowers and beautiful gardens gives great satisfaction both to those who garden and to non-gardeners as well.

However, .there are disadvantages in gardening, particularly for those who suffer with back troubles. More than half the time a person working in a garden is in a bent position. This affects the lower part of the spine. Maintaining this bent position for any length of time interferes with the normal blood circulation, particularly in the legs and head.

Gardening in a small area also restricts walking which is one of the most important types of treatment for afflictions of the lower back and the spinal column.

So, for those people who suffer with back trouble it is important to weigh the advantages and disadvantages of gardening and to use common sense with regard to how much they do.

In any case, all garden lovers or those who garden a lot need regular stretching exercises to counteract the strain from uncomfortable positions and cramped muscles.

Working in a garden has a wonderfully soothing effect on the nervous system, not only for those doing the work but for other members of the family as well. I can still remember the pleasure *I* experienced when my mother-in-law vacated my house to go into the garden!

CHAPTER 10

Massage

The therapeutic benefit of massage has been recognised since ancient times. In spite of the successful cures effected by the use of drugs, in certain countries, massage is still the principal form of treatment used. The use of massage in cases of an injured spinal column, spinal nerves and muscles is of paramount importance, as it is in all cases of locomotor disorders.

The beneficial effects of massage are as follows:

1. It quickens the lymphatic and blood circulation and this leads to increased nutrition of the cells.
2. The pathological products in the damaged cells are dissolved at a greatly increased rate.
3. The elasticity of the cells increases.
4. The muscle tone becomes stronger.
5. The patient has a general feeling of relief because massage relieves the pain.

The basic principles of massage are:

1. Stroking
2. Rubbing
3. Kneading
4. Slapping
5. Vibrating

To carry out a massage it is necessary to have a thorough knowledge of the process and to make absolutely certain that *none of the following conditions are present:*

1. Infectious disease
2. Inflammatory condition of the skin or joints in and around the area to be massaged
3. The body temperature must not be above 37.5°C.
4. Symptoms of thrombosis
5. Internal haemorrhaging
6. Open wound in the massage area
7. Fresh injuries (traumas).

Massage may be carried out at any time and there may be a combination of massage with water and heat as in the case of baths or infra-red light.

Massage has tremendous healing power and also injects fresh power into tired parts of the body, so it has an almost preventative function.

CHAPTER 11

Other forms of treatment

Standard or common forms of treatment of back ache (radiculitis) do not exist. There are many reasons for this.

Although humans are anatomically similar, illnesses and their speed and pattern of development vary greatly among different people. Age and sex make a difference, as do living and working conditions. Diverse, hereditary factors and body resistance must also be taken into account. There are many initial causes of the trouble, and the duration of the illness varies from one person to another. Because of all these factors, a standard method or form of treatment is impractical.

From both the point of view of the patient and the practitioner, a carefully worked out plan of treatment in which both must participate with patience is very difficult to formulate, especially in the case of chronic radiculitis. The "common" forms of treatment for back trouble used by practitioners and specialists are described in previous chapters but there are still some old-fashioned and also relatively new methods which could be used to advantage.

Treatment by hot sand
FOR CHRONIC CASES
Clean, virgin sand from the ocean bed is rich in salt and is quite possibly radioactive. It must be heated to forty-three to fifty-five degrees centigrade and poured into a bath about five to ten centimetres in depth. The patient is buried in this hot sand, leaving the heart region exposed. There must be additional heated covers or blankets for exposed parts. The dry heated sand absorbs the patient's perspiration so that the treatment is easily tolerated.

In a hot climate, sand baths can be taken on the beach in the open air using beach sand heated by the sun. The length of such baths should be from thirty to forty minutes duration.

Clay treatment
FOR CHRONIC CASES
Treatment by hot clay may be the oldest treatment in the world. It

originated in ancient Egypt or Persia and is still used in public baths in villages in Islamic countries. This method is very effective, especially for joint disorders including those involving the spinal column. Clay is well known for its great thermal capacity and low heat conductivity, and it is hydro-absorbent.

Well-crushed clay which has been separated from pebbles is heated in buckets of water to seventy degrees centigrade. After it has been heated the mass is turned out onto boards and enough cold clay is added and mixed to get the right temperature. A "pancake" is then taken from it and placed on the patient's back for a certain length of time — about thirty to forty minutes. It may be placed on the spinal column, legs, the stomach etc. After clay or hot sand treatment a hot shower should be taken.

Treatment by paraffin wax

Paraffin is similar to clay in its thermal capacity and heat conductibility. These properties applied to paraffin make it possible to use it for heat treatment with temperatures up to sixty or seventy degrees centigrade. Although this temperature is somewhat high, it is quite easily tolerated by patients and does not cause burns.

Blocks of paraffin can be put in suitable containers and melted directly over a weak flame or indirectly in hot water. The patient's back is dampened with cold water and then the paraffin is painted on the area with a painter's brush. The paraffin application should be about two centimetres (nearly one inch) thick. Therefore more than one application will probably be needed. After the area to be treated has been "painted" the body must be covered with a plastic sheet and then with a warm blanket. The length of time for the treatment should be from forty to fifty minutes.

Erythema — treatment by burning

FOR ACUTE AND CHRONIC CASES

Erythema is a redness of the skin (a mild form of burning) which is produced by radiation treatment on certain parts of the body with a ray lamp which gives off ultra-violet rays. Treatment is based mainly on the reflex action of the central nervous system but also on the local effects of the rays. This method has been successfully used for many different diseases for a long time in clinics in Eastern Europe and Russia and particularly for the treatment of radiculitis, arthritis and neuritis.

It is better to have this treatment done by a physiotherapist, but if an ultra-violet ray lamp is used at home, *with common sense* then it is quite safe.

During this treatment, the following rules must be observed:

1. Dark glasses should always be worn by both the patient and the person giving the treatment.

2. The necessary dosage must be decided on according to the patient's skin type. Do this by using the following technique: cut out three holes about 13 cm x 13 cm (or 5 in. x 5 in.) on a relatively large sheet of paper and place the paper firmly over the patient's bare stomach. Turn on the lamp and allow it to burn about four or five minutes. After that, focus the lamp over the paper at a height of twenty-five centimetres (ten inches). After one minute cover one hole, after three minutes cover the next hole and in five minutes turn off the lamp. Eight hours after the exposure, look at the skin on the stomach and decide on the exposure which corresponds with the patch of skin that shows a good redness, making sure it is not too pale and not too red. After the choice of the correct dosage, make the first exposure on the most painful area. Most often this is the lower back region, one buttock or the back of the hip. Three days later, do other areas giving a similar dosage of radiation.

3. The approproximate area of the skin burned in the lower region must be 20 × 20 cm (about 8 in. × 8 in.) and on the leg, 20 × 15 cm (about 8 in. × 6 in.).

4. Follow-up treatment may only be given when the redness from the initial exposure has almost disappeared. This will take approximately four to five days depending on the skin type. Dosages of ultra-violet rays for erythema are best repeated two or three times. It is important to note that good results from treatment by burning have also been achieved in arthritic cases.

Banki — suction glasses

This wonderful method of treatment, especially for acute lumbago, muscular rheumatism and for certain ailments of the chest, is completely unknown in many countries. It is used very extensively only in the Slavic countries of Eastern Europe (Russia and Poland) and is called "Banki". In translation this means "cupping".

Banki are found not only in hospitals and doctors' surgeries but in many private houses for family use. During my many years of practising in Germany and in Australia I have often used Banki, (with, of course, the patient's consent). They have been very surprised at the successful results and amazed at the method itself. When first seen, the method of Banki is somewhat frightening to the patient because as well as the small glasses, flame and a fork are necessary parts of the equipment! Naturally a fertile imagination can conjure up untold consequences. However once the method is explained all fears vanish.

An ordinary kitchen fork is used and a thin layer of cotton wool is bound firmly around the prongs. This is then soaked in methylated spirits and then squeezed thoroughly to remove any excess spirit to prevent it from dripping onto the patient's skin.

Next, the part to be treated (back, lower region etc.) is lightly rubbed with vaseline and the patient lies on his stomach. An assistant is necessary to hold the tray containing the small glasses, from twelve to twenty in number, which have smooth rounded edges to avoid cutting into the patient's skin. A lighted match is used to ignite the cotton wool on the fork. Rapidly, one glass after another is taken from the tray. Each time, the flaming fork is held inside the glass for a moment so that the flame consumes the oxygen. This creates a vacuum within the glass. The glass is then immediately placed on the patient's body. The vacuum in the glass sucks in the patient's flesh. Another glass will be applied after the first and so on, until in a few minutes the entire area to be treated is covered with small glasses — this is Banki.

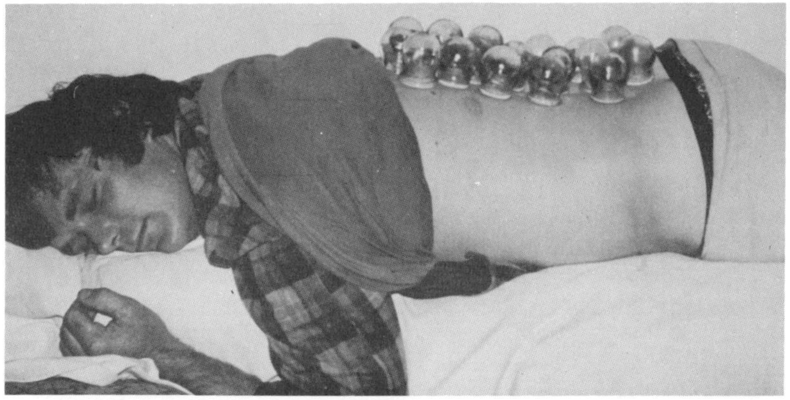

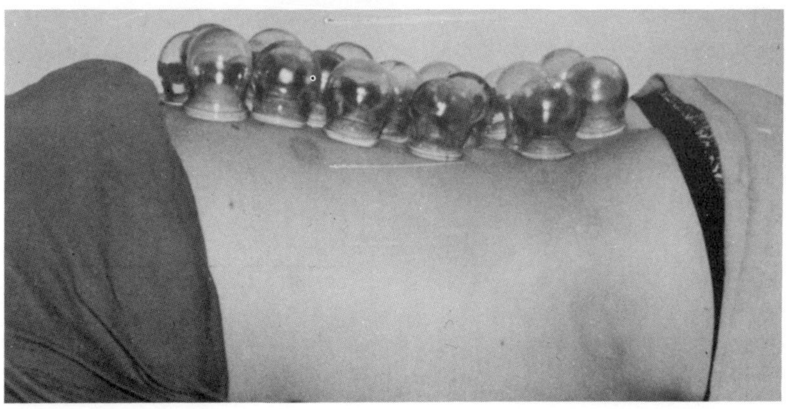

23-24. Banki

The patient experiences a fairly strong pulling feeling of the flesh for about five to ten minutes after which a pleasant feeling of relaxation occurs. When the entire set of glasses has been placed in position, the patient is covered with two or three blankets and is left like this for thirty to forty minutes. The Banki are easily removed by pressing gently on the flesh near the edge of the glass allowing air to penetrate inside and the glass practically falls off. After all the glasses have been removed, the entire area must be rubbed with vaseline. If the Banki have been skilfully applied, a reddish dark-blue ring will show on the flesh. This will disappear completely after a few days.

Banki must be applied only by someone experienced in this method so that the patient or practitioner will not be burnt, or the house set on fire! The proper Banki with wide, blunt rims and rounded bases may be replaced by other small glasses but it is important that the edges are quite blunt and slightly rounded.

The effectiveness of Banki is truly amazing. Someone suffering to such an extent that they are almost doubled over, will, after a short time, perhaps thirty to forty minutes, be able to stand up straight and breathe without pain. It is a sound idea to repeat this treatment in two to three days and of course the patient now has no qualms about the flame and the fork!

What do Banki do?

Apart from the localised effect on the muscles and nerves, the blood supply to that area is increased. They also affect the central nervous system and this eases the contraction of the back muscles.

Treatment by ultra-sound

The first and most important question to be asked is, what is ultra-sound?

With a healthy person the normal ear absorbs a maximum of twenty thousand oscillations in one second. There are noise oscillations very much higher than this, going to hundreds of thousands, even millions, per second, and this is called "ultra-sound". To receive this ultra-sound a special electrical device is used so treatment by ultra-sound has also been included in the chapter dealing with electro-sound, although the character and the operation of the treatment should be bracketed with mechanical therapy.

Treatment by ultra-sound is relatively new. However, there is already a wide scope for its application. It is not only used in medicine but also in agriculture and the fishing industry. Ultra-sound penetrates a person's cells to an approximate depth of five centimetres and sets up a thermal, mechanical, chemical action. The blood supply and the lymphatic drainage of the tissues are considerably increased. In inflamed tissues, acid breakdown products are drained away. Nervous reflexes causing muscle spasms are interrupted which relieves both the spasms and the pain.

Many disorders of the spinal column, both chronic and acute, and injuries, have been successfully treated with the use of ultrasound.

I have used this treatment successfully for more than fifteen years so I know that it can be used by chiropractors as well as physiotherapists.

Treatment by snake and bee venom

Treatment with snake venom called "Viprosit" started about forty years ago in Germany. The most successful and positive results occurred with chronically inflamed spinal nerves and with different types of arthritis. It can be easily understood that the improvement of afflictions of general arthritic conditions will lead on to a general improvement of disorders of the spinal column as its nerves and roots will also improve. This is only logical.

Currently, the practice of using snake and bee venom is widespread in Eastern Europe. Ointments containing these two venoms are popularly used for local applications.

Acupuncture

During the last few years I have often been asked what I think of acupuncture and how effective is it in curing back pains. I can only answer that as yet I have been unable to reach any definite conclusions with regard to this type of treatment.

Treatment by acupuncture is really quite new to doctors of the Western world. We are told that it has been practised in China for over two thousand years. Possibly this method was passed on to the Chinese from Tibet where it was invented by Buddhist monks. Acupuncture only became widely known to the outside world after the Chinese Republic had been established and the once mysterious Tibet became an occupied territory.

Why did we not know about it earlier? For a long time there have been European settlements in China, colonies, concessions, missionary stations. The history and culture of China was studied and yet the world has only just heard about acupuncture! It is hard to say why — perhaps it just suits the leaders to flaunt acupuncture now as an example of the success of their system.

To return to the actual method and result of this treatment: special gold or silver needles, sometimes as thin as cotton, are inserted into carefully chosen places on the body and are left there for specified times. There are more than two hundred such points and apparently these points regulate the function of certain organs. Many doctors have visited China and have seen acupuncture applied. They all confirm that it is quite painless and is so effective as an anaesthetic that complicated operations can be performed.

What are the results of this acupuncture method of treatment on various diseases? As yet there are insufficient positive facts to say that a complete cure of anything is possible.

Pain in the back may be relieved by acupuncture, but I personally doubt whether any kind of radiculitis can be cured by its use.

I think that a variety of treatments, as used in other countries, can be successful when used for the treatment of disorders of the lower part of the spinal column. Paraffin wax, erythema, ultra-sound and Banki particularly need to be added to our list of effective treatments for the lower back.

CHAPTER 12

Self-cure

Self-cure means the cessation of pain (usually sudden pain) without the use of drugs or any medical help. Such cures do occur although they are rare and, to the people concerned, seem to be nothing short of miracles. I know of several such cases and have once had such an experience myself.

I remember that over a period of several days I had my usual lower back pain. Apart from wearing a flannel belt I did not follow any course of treatment. For particular reasons I abstained from taking any pain-killing tablets. In other words, I was doing nothing at all about the pain and was trying to bear my affliction with patience and forbearance as I sat at the table with a pillow behind my back.

I can't remember why I had to leave the table but as I rose from the chair I was suddenly aware of a light, even pleasant, soft "click" in the lower part of my back. At the same moment the pain ceased. I can honestly say that I was surprised by this "miracle". I waited, fearful that the pain would return with increased intensity. It is difficult to believe that for several months I was completely free of all pain.

There was another interesting case involving one of my patients. I received a call from a farm more than 240 kilometres distant telling me that a young woman, her legs "paralysed", was on her way to me. She had been lifting a child when a sudden pain in the back and legs made movement impossible. I do not like cases like this as I think that transportation of patients with badly damaged spinal columns does more harm than good. In these cases I often recommend that the patient be placed in a comfortable position with a low pillow under the head and a smallish pillow under the knees, for about twenty-four to forty-eight hours. It is advisable to give the patient one or two pain-killers and when the pain subsides, to help them have a pleasantly hot bath. Only then, after the pain has subsided, should the patient be moved for treatment.

However, it was too late to give such advice on this occasion as the patient was already on her way. A few hours later a station wagon drew up outside the surgery. The young woman lay in the back on a mattress, her face drawn with pain. There were also two children and a not very robust-looking husband.

The question was — how were we going to get this pain-racked young woman into the surgery without doing more damage or causing more pain. I explained to the husband that I could be of little help because of my own back complaint but he answered with a typical lack of understanding, "Don't worry Doc, she'll be right."

He opened the rear door and began tugging at the mattress on which his wife was lying. When he had managed to get it half-way out, he carefully, I must admit, turned his wife onto her right side and then clasping her round the waist, tried to stand her on her feet. What followed is now rather a blurred memory but I do remember one agonised shriek from the woman as she and her husband both fell on the lawn in a mass of tangled arms and legs. What followed next was so unexpected and so astonishing that it left an indelible impression on my mind. The young woman, without help, stood up and walked into the surgery as if nothing untoward had happened.

"I'm all right, I'm all right," she kept saying. "The pain has gone." And she *was* all right.

The "miracle" had happened. She required no manipulation or other treatment. I simply put a hot German plaster on her back, gave her a fairly large amount of sodium salicylate and made her comfortable on the surgery couch where she rested for about an hour.

There is one final "miracle cure" case I should like to mention. I didn't actually see it happen myself but the account was given to me by a Polish acquaintance who was an ex-soldier. Like thousands of other migrants he worked as a manual labourer and in the course of his work, he often shifted without help heavy railway sleepers. On one occasion when he and another man were working together, he suddenly felt sharp pains in the lower part of his back and he slipped and almost fell. "My feet felt as if they didn't belong to me," he said.

He was taken by ambulance to the hospital in a nearby country town. He was given a pain-killing injection by the doctor and X-rays of his back were taken after which the doctor recommended that he should be placed in traction. He didn't know how heavy the weight on his leg was but he remembers that only the injections lessened the pain.

Being new to the country and its ways he was embarrassed by his helplessness and the fact that he could not go to the toilet on his own but had to call a nurse to bring him a bottle whenever it was necessary. On the second night when he needed a bedpan and he rang the bell, the nurse brought him a bottle. He did not know the language and his embarrassment increased as he didn't know what signs to make to show that he wanted a bedpan and not just a bottle. He decided he would have to wait until an orderly arrived in the morning to attend to his needs. But Nature isn't always so accommodating.

You can perhaps imagine the mental state of this man. Once he had been a proud and respected citizen in his own country and here he was, an alien in an alien land, a manual labourer with not even enough words of his new tongue to ask for a bedpan and he was about to disgrace himself, as he thought, by soiling his bed. This could not be allowed to happen.

Gathering all his strength, he somehow managed to free himself from the traction, pulled himself off the bed and rushed quickly as he could to the toilet.

"Mission accomplished", he felt an inward glow of satisfaction as he returned to the room and he found that all his back pain had disappeared. He was discharged from the hospital the next day and six years later when he was telling me the story there still had been no recurrence of the pain.

These almost miraculous "instant" cures are rare. They are always viewed with awe and wonder by the people concerned. And it is understandable that they are often regarded with suspicion and disbelief by many people, as there seems to be no proven scientific explanation for them. Therefore, they puzzle the medical men and excite the imagination of the ordinary person. Miracles do exist in Nature but the supreme miracle is the human body itself — the way it is built and the way in which it functions.

It is still a mystery why a suddenly healthy body succumbs to disease or how certain unhealthy conditions arise. Similarly, there is no known explanation for sudden cures, from the disappearance of warts to the disappearance of the dreaded cancer. They are riddles which continue to baffle medical science but provide rich bonuses for the persons involved.

To explain why there were cures in the three cases I have cited is not easy. However, in these instances, and, being thoroughly familiar with the anatomy of the spinal column, it is logical to suppose that because of the physical exertion incurred, there was a flattening and slipping of the intervertebral discs, which lessened the compression of the roots of the spinal cord that had been causing such agonising pain and, in some cases, had "paralysed" the legs. In the last two cases, the effect was similar to the manipulation done by chiropractors. These movements widened the spaces between the vertebrae and the discs returned to their normal positions and ceased pressing on the roots of the spinal cord.

But, of course, this is only supposition!

CHAPTER 13

Twelve rules for lifting

The incorrect lifting of heavy loads and the carrying of them in awkward positions are two main causes of injury to the spinal column, particularly to the lower region.

Through observation of many hundreds of patients in my practice I know that over half the number of lower spinal injuries are due to lack of knowledge of the rules concerning the lifting of weights. Knowledge of the correct rules for weight-lifting has a significant bearing on the prevention of back injury and on aggravation of an already injured back.

Twelve rules for lifting and carrying loads

1. Never attempt to lift and carry loads beyond your own strength.
2. Always face the object to be lifted squarely, face on.
3. Stand as close to the object as possible.
4. Spread your legs apart, at least the same width as will match the width of your shoulders. Make sure that both feet are flat on the ground and that both feet are standing on the same elevation.
5. Bend your legs slightly at the knees.
6. Keep the spinal column as straight as possible.
7. Never bend only the lower back, but bend *both* the hips and the *knees.*
8. Just as professional weight-lifters do, *before* you commence to lift, take a deep breath. This action reduces the pressure from outside.
9. Regardless of how light the object is, never lift it suddenly or with a jerk.
10. Never attempt by yourself to lift any heavy object above your waist.
11. Always hold the object with the entire palm and not just with the fingers.
12. Avoid carrying unbalanced loads and always hold the object as close to the body as possible.

These rules may seem unnecessary but scientific experiments have proved that with the incorrect lifting of a weight, when the spinal column is in the bent position, the pressure on the base of the spine is approximately ten times greater than the weight of the object being lifted. As an example: if a farmer lifts a bag of superphosphate weighing eighty-two kilos, and he lifts it in an incorrect manner, the pressure on the lower part of the spine will be equal to eight hundred and twenty kilos *plus* the weight of the upper part of his body.

It is not difficult to imagine the extent of possible injury to the intervertebral discs, the joints, nerve roots and muscles, particularly to a person not accustomed to physical work. And it is important to remember that heavy or overweight men are more susceptible to back strain as there is greater pressure on the lower part of the spine when they straighten up after a heavy lifting.

Women

Women are much more susceptible to back injuries than men because their entire muscular system is weaker than that of men, and the whole cartilaginous system is likewise weaker. Women usually sustain their back injuries during everyday household chores: lifting a basket of laundry, making a bed, working in the garden or lifting children. Surprisingly, the percentage of lower back injuries in women is not as high as that of injuries to the neck and upper rib cage.

In any case, in Australia and in some European countries, industrial laws prohibit women from lifting weights of more than sixteen kilos and objects to be lifted may not exceed four and a half kilos if they are to be raised to a height of more than two metres.

CHAPTER 14

Correct body position and supports

What is the best type of bed for a sore back? is a question asked regularly by my patients.

One would think there is only one logical answer to this question: "One in which you feel comfortable and sleep well." But this answer is only partially correct, for the following reasons.

Suppose that a normal, healthy person is used to sleeping in a particular bed, soft, warm, having perhaps an air or water mattress and the comfort of an eiderdown or an electric blanket. The body will grow accustomed to these luxuries even if they are considered unnecessary and unhealthy by some standards.

Undoubtedly such people will sleep well and feel very comfortable — when they are not sick. However, they will have a significantly greater chance of suffering if they develop back trouble than the person who sleeps in what might be termed a more Spartan fashion.

In this respect some parents make a serious mistake out of love for their children by giving them beds that are too soft and cosy.

FOR HEALTHY PEOPLE WANTING TO PREVENT SPINAL ILLNESSES a good brand of firm spring mattress is required. It is not necessary to sleep on the floor or on boards, but if the mattress is not sufficiently firm it may be necessary to place boards underneath. Pillows should be comfortable but not too high.

The most relaxed position for the body is lying flat on the back but this is not necessary for everyone.

IF A PERSON ALREADY HAS A HISTORY OF SPINAL PROBLEMS, then sleeping on a flat and hard bed is incorrect as this will only increase the chance of a recurrence of the trouble and each new bout tends to make the person's condition worse. I also recommend that people in this category sleep in single beds.

FOR PEOPLE ACTUALLY SUFFERING FROM SPINAL ILLNESS, it is imperative to provide the greatest amount of comfort.

This also applies to people with chronic spinal deformities.

Naturally such people will require a soft mattress that will mould itself to the contours of the back. The bed must be warm (never cold) and a single bed is essential.

In this last group I would include ageing and very old people. To clarify the last statement let me tell about one couple I had to deal with.

He was suffering from severe osteoarthritis of the spine and she was a solidly built and physically healthy woman. Before he finished his course of treatment he asked me what type of mattress I would recommend for him. I explained everything that was necessary for him to know and then I added, "And it will be better if you sleep in a bed on your own". His wife, who was with him suddenly said in a complaining voice, "And what about my cold feet?"

"You will have to buy bed socks Madam," I replied firmly.

How to sit down

Many people spend more than half their lives in a sitting position. This is particularly the case in large towns. They sit at work and they sit in a car for perhaps one or two hours, going to and from work.

Millions of people spend from six to eight hours in offices. Returning home, they sit down to eat. Afterwards they relax watching television, talking, or indulging in hobbies from cards to crochet, still sitting down. On days off or on the weekends their relaxation and pleasure is driving somewhere but rarely, if ever, walking.

In a sitting position, the lower region of the back bears twice as much pressure as when it is in a standing position. The discs in particular are subjected to a great deal of pressure if the positions of the spine and/or the legs, are incorrect. With continued sitting there is a weakening due to tiredness of the back muscles. The spinal column gradually slumps and harmful effects on the spinal column are greatly increased.

Long periods of sitting are particularly harmful to people who already suffer with pain in the lower region of the back.

Not only from an aesthetic but also from a physical point of view, it is very necessary to position the body correctly, when sitting down.

One should always sit up straight, preferably leaning against the back of the chair. Do not sit on the edge like a chicken on a perch. When driving long distances in a car be sure that the back of the seat gives full support to the whole body or it will be very uncomfortable. If necessary, place a cushion in the small of the back. It is very important to sit close to the wheel and still be seated comfortably. This is particularly important for truck drivers or grader and tractor drivers. With long-distance driving it is a good idea to stop the car once in a while, get out and stretch the muscles by walking round for a moment and doing a few simple exercises for the legs and back. These little breaks will be of tremendous benefit.

When sitting, the feet must touch the floor or ground and it is best if they are positioned parallel to each other. If the legs and feet are in the correct position when you are sitting down, then the pressure on the lumbar region of the back is greatly reduced. Crossing the legs or placing one on the other for long periods is not recommended. This is not only bad for the spine it also affects the blood circulation in the lower limbs.

Corsets

The use of corsets for support and for maintaining the correct position of the spinal column is quite common. I should say that it is practised more often than is necessary and often without first consulting an orthopaedic specialist. It must always be remembered that the *best support for the spinal column is strong well-developed back and stomach muscles.* They can be kept strong and in good condition by special exercises.

The frequent wearing of a corset weakens the muscles and makes them "lazy". It may support the spinal column but when it fits tightly round the body it adversely affects the functioning of the internal organs. For elderly people it is particularly unhealthy to wear corsets as the functions of their internal organs could be disturbed.

During my practising years I recommended the wearing of corsets as a temporary measure only and then for particular people, mostly men working on graders and tractors, and for those who went horse back riding.

There are many types of corsets but they can be divided basically into two groups: hard and soft.

I repeat, that corsets should be worn only after consulting an orthopaedic specialist.

Belts

In contrast to corsets, belts do not give support but only keep the lower part of the back warm and protect it from being cold and getting chills, particularly for outdoor workers like shearers, brick layers, carpenters, and road workers. Anyone working in draughty conditions or cold weather, especially in the winter time, will benefit from wearing a belt.

Anyone can make one of these belts by using some coloured flannel. It is better to wear the belt over a garment, rather than next to the skin, and it is advisable to have a spare one.

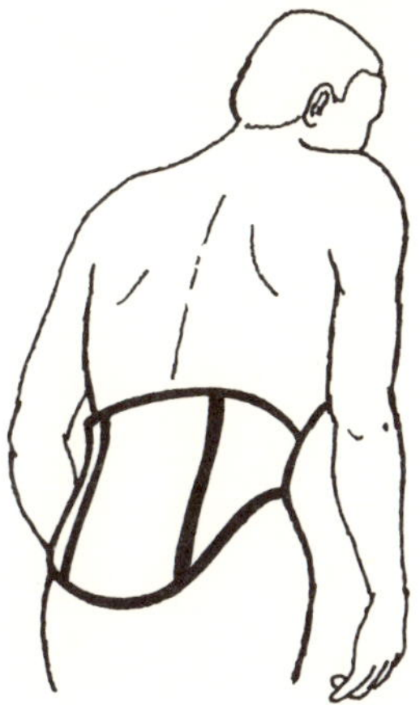

25. *"Shearer Master" red flannel belt*

Excellent red flannel belts are available.* There are also leather belts of varying widths. These are usually worn by men lifting heavy weights or by sportsmen, weight-lifters, wrestlers and people involved in hard physical labour. For other occupations, such belts have no practical value.

In addition there are many types of elastic belts which are sometimes used by certain people.

*"Shearer Master" red flannel belts may be bought from Melro, 411 Sussex Street Sydney.

CHAPTER 15

Rules to live by

Preventative measures can be divided into two groups:
1. Those for people who have a past history of lower spinal pain or injury, or who are suffering present discomfort.
2. Those for people who have never suffered with lower back injury or pain.

There is a vital difference between these measures in that the former group must be aware of and must always remember and follow carefully all the safety measures already emphasised. If they neglect to follow the instructions given, there is every reason to expect a recurrence and an intensification of their past condition.

The second group is more fortunate and must concentrate on the preventative measures which are devised, in the main, for the most susceptible areas of the spinal column.

People of the first group must learn to live with the fact that they have a weak place in the lower part of the spinal column which may, at any moment, sometimes without warning and for no apparent reason "knock them down". For these people, regardless of the form of treatment to be given or where it takes place, no guarantee can ever be given that the ailment will be permanently or completely cured.

So, if you have had trouble with the lower part of the back, it is well to remember that it may recur at any time and therefore preventative measures are particularly important for you.

1. Try to avoid sudden movements or any knocks, long-term vibrations of the back, (horse riding, tractor driving, bulldozer driving, truck driving, or travelling on corrugated or rough roads).

2. Avoid frequent or sudden turns of the torso, especially in the same direction repeatedly. Also avoid, if possible, keeping the body in a bent or twisted position for any length of time, especially for a prolonged period.

3. Avoid lifting heavy weights. If it is necessary to lift them, remember the rules (see Chapter 13).

4. Avoid running and jumping.

5. Never sit on wet ground or cold rocks (as you may well do if you are picnicking or bush walking). Always remove wet clothing as soon as possible. It has already been suggested that allowing a bathing suit to dry on one's body is not a good idea for "back sufferers".

6. Don't allow the whole body to become chilled, particularly the lower back and legs.

7. During the cold months of the year always wear warm underclothing and a flannel back belt around the lower back.

8. During the cold months of the year, don't get into a cold bed. Immediately you get into a cold bed, your body temperature drops and this affects the spinal roots. Use an electric blanket, a hot water bottle, even a hot brick or sand or an ordinary bottle filled with hot water to warm the bed.

9. In the summertime, "sunbake" the lower part of the body but do not expose it to the wind.

10. Never neglect the daily exercise routine. But remember not to do it after a meal or before sleeping. Exercises will develop elasticity in the lower part of the back and will prevent the pinching of roots and nerves as well as stopping the joining vertebrae from growing together (locking). It also strengthens the muscles needed for correct posture.

11. Avoid coughing and constipation, or do something to remedy these two conditions, as straining and pressure from them may provoke pain in the back.

12. If at any moment during a working period you suddenly become conscious that your back is beginning to ache, do something else for a short time or have a brief complete rest.

13. Periodically, take large doses of Vitamin B1 as it raises the resistance of the spinal cord, spinal roots and its nerves.

For those fortunate people of the second group, preventative measures consist exclusively of building up the resistance of the lower part of the spine.

1. Systematic walking and daily exercises must be undertaken for the maintenance and development of elasticity and flexibility of the spinal column.

2. Strictly observe all the rules for the correct lifting and carrying of weights.

3. Regulate physical strain by alternating the routine of heavy strain with lighter tasks.
4. Avoid draughts. Avoid over-chilling the back.
5. Try to remember that as surely as you think, "It can't happen to me" then, unhappy reader, I have no doubt that *you* will be a lower lumbar trouble victim.

＃ CHAPTER 16

Lubrication

Nearly everyone knows the story of *The Wizard of Oz* made familiar to millions of people all over the world through the acting of the unforgettable Judy Garland. For those younger people who didn't have the joy of seeing the picture or who don't know the story, let me re-cap one part as it is so relevant to the subject about which I am writing.

The little girl in the story met a man made of tin. As the story unfolds, the tin woodsman, after a year of exposure in the forest, could not move because his joints were so rusty. Our little girl, Dorothy, oiled his rusty joints and he was then able to travel on with her to see the wonderful Wizard of Oz.

I'm sure that as you read the following pages you will understand how perfectly this illustrates and emphasises this important point I want to make.

Of the many different conditions that affect the spinal column, particularly the lower region, arthritic radiculitis would probably be the most prevalent.

Millions of people in every country in the world suffer from this painful and crippling disease and many millions of dollars have been spent in researching its origin, in providing relief and in searching for a cure for these sufferers.

It is mainly osteoarthritis which affects the spinal column. However it is not widely known that gout arthritis is far from being a rare condition and medical statistics suggest that one out of every four or five people has symptoms of this type of arthritis after the age of forty-five or fifty.

The reasons for this may be the excessive eating of meat, particularly in Australia (and in other Western countries where the standard of living is high) as well as the excessive consumption of alcohol, particularly beer.

Why does arthritis develop?

Is it hereditary?

Could climatic conditions be a factor?

Is it because of a person's work?

Is it because of the type of food we eat?

Medical science has not yet established any one particular

reason or factor and at this point of time there are no reliable methods for effecting a complete cure of this prevalent and crippling condition. Yet unfortunately, osteoarthritis of the spinal column is a common occurrence and it causes dramatic changes in the spinal column.

The first change is when the joints become dry and there is a calcification of the intervertebral discs. Then spurs form on the corners of the vertebrae and gradually fuse together so that the spinal column begins to resemble a stick of very old bamboo.

Next, movements become extremely painful and restricted and in some cases are almost completely impossible. The lower part of the body can barely be moved and to turn the head, the entire body must be moved.

However strange it may seem, it often happens that osteoarthritis affects the spinal column alone and leaves the rest of the body's joints untouched.

In 1957, D.D. Alexander, after studying arthritis and its subsequent effects, published a book, entitled *Arthritis and Common Sense.* His theory is that, and I quote: "Arthritis is a deficiency of specific dietary oils. This deficiency results in lack of better grade lubricating oil for the body joints."

He compiled diets rich in Vitamin D for those suffering from arthritis, which included as many as five eggs a day. Alexander also insisted on the regular intake of plain cod liver oil, saying that, and again I quote: "cod liver oil is a key weapon against arthritis". According to him, even lumbago is the result of a lack of lubrication on the roots of the spinal cord.

Treatment of many diseases with cod liver oil and the intake of food rich in Vitamin D was undertaken for hundreds of years before Alexander wrote his book, so his theory was far from new. What was new was the idea that the intake of cod liver oil and the foods rich in Vitamin D *could* lubricate the joints.

This idea may have a positive application for the treatment of people under forty-five years of age or so, particularly children, and for those with a normal cholesterol content in their blood. Alexander's book was welcomed by millions of osteoarthritic sufferers, many of whom began taking large doses of cod liver oil and maintained the intake over a long period. If they were not cured, at least they received some relief from the arthritic pain. This was particularly so where children were affected.

The intake of cod liver oil also made joint movements easier for older people but, in addition, it had the very adverse effect of helping them to die sooner than necessary.

Unhappily there is an irrefutable fact established by medical science: Vitamin D, which is found in abundance in cod liver oil, facilitates the rise of a substance in the blood called cholesterol. Cholesterol is stored in the form of slimy plates on the walls of the blood vessels, causing blockages, which in turn lead to heart disease and strokes.

Alexander's diets, which sometimes included five eggs a day were not helpful to elderly people because of the cholesterol-forming yolks. Apart from this, the systematic intake of plain cod liver oil in large doses cannot be tolerated by the stomach and liver of an older person.

The idea of lubrication for the thinner (dry) type of body, as opposed to those with a more fatty covering, is wonderful and very important. Lubrication can help all the joints, including the joints of the spinal column. However, for those people inclined to be overweight, or even "comfortably" covered, I would suggest as a substitute for cod liver oil maize oil or sunflower oil, and in considerably smaller quantities.

The table below indicates the high content of cholesterol in egg yolk and cod liver oil. As can be seen, they stand in second and third places in the following table.

CHOLESTEROL CONTENT IN FOOD PRODUCTS IN MILLIGRAMS PER 100 GRAMS OF RAW PRODUCTS

Brain	1810
Egg yolk	1560
Cod liver oil	570
Kidneys	365
Liver — pork	340
Liver — beef	265
Butter	244
Margarine	186
Dripping	122
Chicken	113
Veal	84
Beef	67
Pork	60
Milk (non-skim)	13.4
Milk (skim)	2.8

CHAPTER 17

Fasting

The most effective treatment for those people who are overweight is fasting. Before discussing this most important method of treatment, it is interesting to delve into its history, the roots of which go back to the pre-Christian era.

More than two thousand years ago, Greek physicians and philosophers noted the beneficial effects of fasting on the individual. Four hundred years before the birth of Christ, Hippocrates, the "father of medicine", and later, Asclepias, founded the first-known school of physicians in Rome. Here, fasting as a form of treatment was recommended in preference to medicine.

In the first century of the Christian era, Galen was in favour of this method. The great Arab physician, Avicenna, who lived in the tenth century, also advocated treatment through nutritional methods and often treated his patients by starving them. Most people know that Christ fasted in the wilderness for forty days and the treatment of illness through fasting is mentioned many times in the Bible and also in the Talmud.

Complete or partial fasting is still practised as part of religious rituals and at certain set times by adherents of the three most popular religions of the world, Christianity, Buddhism and Mohammedanism. Followers of Islam fast during the day for Ramadan which is the ninth month of their calendar year.

As a general rule, people who fast regularly for religious reasons, Orthodox Russians for example, are less prone to disease and also have a longer life span.

The history of medicine can produce many other examples of treatment by fasting, however, I don't want to enlarge further on this fascinating subject, except to mention two famous names familiar to most of the present readers, Gandhi and Bernard Shaw.

Mahatma Gandhi, the spiritual leader of India, was in his hundredth year when an assassin ended his life. He was noted for his moderation in eating and his long periods of fasting, although it must be admitted that they were mostly politically motivated. In his memoirs, Gandhi recommended fasting, not only for purifying the body, but as a way of developing the mental and spiritual capacities of the mind.

Shaw was a giant among the writers and philosophers of his time but few people know that he considered that his voluntary days of fasting contributed to his prodigious output of writing and also to his long and active life.

All of us would be appalled at the thought of impending starvation, particularly those who over-eat. And prolonged lack of food will indeed finally make the body sick and death will follow. Unhappily, I have seen this happen to hundreds of people in my lifetime, particularly during the last war. Yet heart trouble, diseases of the liver and stomach, arthritis and psychiatric and nervous illnesses all may be treated through fasting. Overweight responds very successfully to diet and fasting. Complete or partial fasting, if carried out sensibly and correctly, may not only greatly benefit a person by preventing or helping to cure an illness, it may also increase the life span considerably and that is something mankind has always wanted.

What occurs during fasting?

If we abstain from food for a period of time, the energy used for the digestive and absorption processes can be used in cleansing the body of the poison substances that accumulate. Waste — slag — which gradually accumulates, acts like a poison in the body, and it will be more quickly passed out of it. Fats will dissolve more speedily and weight will decrease.

Short term fasting is advantageous to all the organs of the system. The stomach and the intestines are the first to benefit and then the liver and nervous system.

During fasting days, the entire organic system is able to rest, after which it functions with greater efficiency.

Types of fasting

COMPLETE FASTING

Complete fasting may only be carried out if the following rules are strictly adhered to and it should be of no longer duration than two to three days. Any period of fasting that extends longer than three days should be spent in hospital and under the surveillance of a doctor.

1. During complete fasting, do not take any food at all but it is vitally necessary to drink unlimited quantities of hot water with honey. Up to eight tablespoons of honey are allowed per day.

2. Avoid physical activity during the fasting period.

3. Keep the body warm but do not overheat it by lying in the sun or by taking hot baths or showers.

4. Avoid alcohol and keep smoking to a minimum.

5. As actual bodily weakness increases and there is an awareness of a lack of strength, two to three cups of coffee may be taken during the day.

6. After the fasting period ends, normal meals should be resumed very gradually.

PARTIAL FASTING

Partial fasting involves abstinence from food for a limited number of hours only. Perhaps from five to ten but certainly not less than five.

In this instance, avoid food that contains starch, such as bread, rice, macaroni, vermicelli and potatoes. It is also very important *not* to overload the stomach with too much food immediately after fasting. This point must be emphasised as a person feeling hungry is very likely to overeat at the first opportunity. For example, if partial fasting has been carried out for five hours (from 8 a.m. until 1 p.m.) then it is advisable to have one or two light meals at intervals between 1 p.m. and retiring for the night.

If fasting has continued for ten hours (from 8 a.m. until 6 p.m.) have one light meal before going to bed.

Drinking hot water with honey is permitted as in complete fasting. Partial fasting for a period of from three to five days may be done at home without medical supervision.

COMBINED TYPES OF FASTING

Combined fasting is a combination of partial fasting (limited to a few hours) followed by a relief day. A relief day is a period from 8 a.m. one day until 8 a.m. the following day during which only fresh fruits (with the exception of bananas) and vegetables may be eaten but in unlimited quantities. Fruit juices should be the only beverage taken.

Fruits: Apples, pears, citrus fruits, stone fruits, strawberries. All are suitable.

Vegetables: Tomatoes, cucumbers, lettuce, carrots, cabbage, rock melons and water melons. There is a large variety from which to choose.

If there is a need or craving for liquids other than fruit juices, three cups of black coffee without sugar are permitted.

How often should we fast and which of the above-listed methods is most likely to help with weight loss? From my own experience in observing patients over a long period of time, I would recommend more frequent use of the partial fasting method than the occasional long or complete fast. In this way, a steady weight loss without harm may be gradually achieved.

To summarise, these are the conditions which *must* be observed with all types of fasting.

1. Take a dose of any laxative in the evening at the beginning of the fasting period.
2. During the fasting period do not indulge in any type of hard physical activity.
3. Keep the body warm but not overheated.
4. Drink lots of hot water with honey.
5. Don't drink alcohol.
6. Smoke less.
7. As strength lessens, lie down and rest more often.
8. At the end of the fast, take small amounts of food only and very slowly build up to the normal intake.

Don't be afraid to fast. The benefits of fasting are well worth the effort. Sensible and systematic fasting combined with relief days will help to cure minor ills, bring beneficial results to your whole system, prolong life and give you a sense of well-being and joy.

The last word

Having finished this manuscript, I read it through as a complete work as if I were reading it for the first time. When I came to the last page I reviewed it objectively (if an author ever can be objective about his own writing) and I felt something was missing. What was it? What had I neglected to say, to explain, to describe, more clearly?

This subject has been a part of me for practically my whole life. I thought I knew, from my study and my experience, every facet of my specialised subject. I thought it was all an open book to me. And I had endeavoured to pass on the benefit of my knowledge and work to my readers.

But somehow I felt I had failed in my objective. I couldn't sleep that night. Next day I re-read all that I had written and my doubts and misgivings only increased. The more I thought about it, the less satisfied I was.

As I sat there wondering where I had failed, almost without any conscious motivation on my part, thoughts of people who had touched my life at some point in time started to drift across my mind's eye like a moving picture. Ah, yes. There was Sister Alicia! Suddenly the missing piece of the jigsaw fell neatly into place. It was just a text book I had written and that was not my original intention.

I wanted to help people with the medical experience and training I had had, but I wanted this book to be a "human" one and not merely a factual work. There must be people in my book. And so this "last word" was born.

Let me begin my story just thirty years ago which was when I arrived in Australia with my wife and my two boys.

My experiences as a doctor were wide and had varied from the normal to the bizarre as any medical man with a war time practice behind him would know. I had already had some scientific works published in Germany and my practical medical experience had been greater than most doctors of my age (which was forty-two).

However all this was of no avail to me in Australia. I was sent to an army camp to wash the dishes and be a kitchen hand. With me was another young European doctor and together we washed dishes. We worked very well in our new sphere from early morning until late at night with a short midday break. Our living quarters were in a nearby barracks. I can never forget those dishes, those grease-covered frying pans and saucepans, the large heavy milk cans. And the mountains of dirty plates.

The days passed into weeks and still we washed dishes. Our hands roughened and our brains seemed to atrophy doing this "medical" work but my colleague and I worked on meticulously and without complaint, as doctors do with their duties.

One day after lifting a heavy milk can I aggravated an old back injury and found myself in hospital. For three days and three nights the duty sister administered some pain-killers. No physician came to examine me as I had no particular doctor for whom I could ask. I was just a "Mr Nobody", a stranger in an alien land. There was not even the comfort of a friend to help me and the iron barrier of language shut me away from those about me. It was less than two months since our arrival on the first transport ship and my vocabulary was limited to a few simple phrases. I hadn't even learnt to swear! Just a little sympathy at such a time means so much to a lonely stranger.

I was a man with a long, incomprehensible name which Australians couldn't even begin to say. I was one of those "reffos" flooding into the country, about to "rob Australians of work" — washing greasy dishes, perhaps!

The future looked grim indeed. My hopes for our new life wavered to a pessimistic low. What if my health failed? What was going to happen to my family? Naturally all this anxiety had an adverse effect on my physical condition.

On one of the darkest days of this period of my life, I met a Catholic nun, Sister Alicia. She was of medium height, with a pleasant round face and deep-set eyes. She was visiting patients and finally she stopped by my bed. It must have been the sight of me that made her linger. I was obviously in great pain and I suppose I looked exhausted, as I was after so many sleepless nights. I hadn't shaved for days and perhaps my derelict appearance aroused a special pity in her for me.

She spoke to me but I could only shake my head uncomprehendingly. She sat down on the side of the bed and took my hand in her own firm round little hands, closed her eyes and began to pray. It was as if some warm invisible current passed from those hands and flowed gently into me and I too closed my eyes and called to God for help. We were of different religious faiths, complete strangers and yet here we were, talking to the same God. It was very soon after her visit that I knew I had turned the corner.

For the first time since I had entered the hospital I slept soundly through the whole night and a few days later I was discharged from the hospital.

I remember a wonderful man, a French-American surgeon and philosopher, Alexis Karrel, who wrote in one of his books about the power and mystery of prayer. Can we ever solve the mystery of the healing power of prayer? If it is truly sincere, this power is enormous. Karrel also says that praying for another is even more fruitful than for one's self.

And here, as I end my book, I am not ashamed to say, that when all my scientific knowledge and my use of known treatments have failed, I too, have prayed for many of my patients.

Explanation of the terms used

Abdomen   The portion of the body lying between the thorax and the pelvis

Abdominal   Pertaining to the abdomen

Aesthetics   Belonging to the appreciation of the beautiful (good taste)

Agony   Absence of sensibility due to pain

Anatomy   The science of bodily structure

Arthritis   Any joint inflammation

Atrophy   Degeneration of the cells

Balneology   Science of baths

Balneotherapy   Treatment of disease with baths

Cartilage   The gristle or white elastic substance attached to articular bone surfaces and forming parts of the skeleton

Calcification   Deposition of calcium salts in the tissues

Cervical   Pertaining to the neck

Chronic   Long continued

Coccyx   Small triangular bone ending spinal column in man

Compression   Abnormal pressure upon the brain

Congenital   Existing at or before birth

Contraction   A drawing together; a shortening or shrinkage

Deformation   Change for the worse

Degeneration   Alteration of tissue from a higher to a lower form

Dehydration   The removal of water from a substance

Disc   Intervertebral. The layer of fibro-cartilage between the bodies of adjoining vertebrae

Diabetes   Disease with excessive glucose-charged urine

Dorsal   Pertaining to the back

Erythema   Redness of skin

Evolution   Developing from a pre-existing form

Excretory system   System which expels waste from the body

Fibrous   Composed of, or containing, fibres

Fracture   The breaking of a bone

Genetic   Pertaining to reproduction

Genital organs   Those organs pertaining to reproduction

Gibbon   Indian anthropoid ape, with very long arms and without a tail

Gout   Disease with joint inflammation and chalky deposits due to disturbance of purine metabolism of the body

Gynaecology   The branch of medicine which is concerned with diseases of women

Hereditary   Descending by inheritance; transmitted from one generation to another

Immunity   Protection against any particular disease

Impulse   Impelling push

Intervertebral   Situated between vertebrae

Lateral   Pertaining to a side

Ligament   Strong fibrous bands which bind and hold the bones in position

Locomotor disorder   Movement disorder

Lumbar puncture   The tapping of the spinal membranes in the lumbar region

Lumbar region   or lower spine

Lumbago   Muscles and joints affected by contraction

Lumbo-sacral   The region of the lumbar spine and the sacral spine, or more particularly the junction of the last lumbar vertebra and the sacrum

Lymphatic system   The lymphatic glands, vessels, spaces, sinuses, and lacteals collectively

Menopause   Period when menstruation ceases

Metabolic   Process, in an organism or single cell, by which nutritive material is built up into living matter or protoplasm is broken down into simpler substances

Muscle tone   The condition of a slight but continuous contraction in muscle; a sign of good health

Neurology   Science of disorder of the nerves

Orthopaedic   That branch of surgery which deals with the correction of deformities and with the treatment of chronic disease of the joints and spine

Os   Bone (Latin)

Osteoarthritis   Multiple degenerative joint disease

Ovary   The female gland in which ova are formed

Oxydesis   The acid binding power, especially of the blood

Paralytic   Pertaining to, or affected with, paralysis

Pathological   Abnormal; not normal

Physiology   Science of normal functions

Physiotherapy   Treatment of disease by natural forces, such as light, heat, air, water etc.

Pigment   Natural colouring-matter of a tissue

Pine needle extract   Extract made from pine oil

Poliomyelitis   Inflammation of grey substance of spinal cord

Posterior   Situated behind or toward the rear

Prostate   A gland surrounding the neck of the bladder and urethra in the male

Psychological   Mental branch of science which treats the mind and mental processes

Radiculitis   Inflammation of the nerve roots

Radix   For spinal root (Latin)

Reflex   Action which is independent of the will

Reproductive system   The fusion of a male sexual cell with a female sexual cell

Rheumatic   Pertaining to, or affected with, rheumatism

Rickets   A deficiency disease of infancy and childhood in which the normal process of ossification is disturbed; the bones become crooked and deformed

Roots of spine cord — (Radix)   Spinal ganglia

Rupture   The bursting or breaking of a part

Sacrum   The triangular bone between and behind the two ilia

Sciatica   Neuralgia and neuritis of the sciatic nerve

Sciatic nerve   The largest nerve in the body; begins in the sacral region

Scoliosis   Curve from side to side situated about the middle of the back, sometimes with pronounced drooping of shoulder

Sinus   An air cavity in one of the cranial bones (accessory sinus of the nose)

Slipped disc   An intervertebral disc that has been forced or squeezed out of position

Spa resort   Place where there is a mineral spring

Spasm   A sudden violent, involuntary contraction

Spina bifida   Congenital cleft of vertebral column

Spinal column   A supporting part of the skeleton consisting of vertebrae

Spinal cord   The nerve structure occupying the vertebral canal

Stock salt   Salt which farmers use for their animals

Symptoms   Sign or token of the existence of something

Tendon   The fibrous cord by which a muscle is attached

Therapeutic   The treatment of disease

Thrombosis   Coagulation of blood in blood vessel or organ

Thoracic   Of, or pertaining to, the chest

Tissue   An aggregation of fibres and cells composing a structural element

Tonsillitis   Inflammation of a tonsil

Trauma   A wound or injury

Tumour   Local swelling from a growth

Ultra-violet ray   Invisible rays of the spectrum

Uric acid   A crystalline acid found in urine and in some organs of the body

Varicose vein   A greatly enlarged and contorted vein

Venom   A poison produced by snake and bee

Vertebra   One of the bones forming the spinal column

Notes

Notes

Notes

Notes

Notes

Notes